THE ORIGINS OF
Ventricular Arrhythmias

Using the ECG as a Key Tool for Localization

ONLINE ACCESS

The purchase of a new copy of this book entitles the first retail purchaser to free personal online access to a digital version of this edition.

Please send a copy of your purchase receipt to info@cardiotext.com with subject BOGUN EBOOK, and we will email you a redemption code along with instructions on how to access the digital file.

THE ORIGINS OF
Ventricular Arrhythmias

Using the ECG as a Key Tool for Localization

Frank M. Bogun, MD, FACC
Professor of Internal Medicine
Section of Cardiac Electrophysiology
Division of Cardiovascular Medicine
University of Michigan
Ann Arbor, Michigan

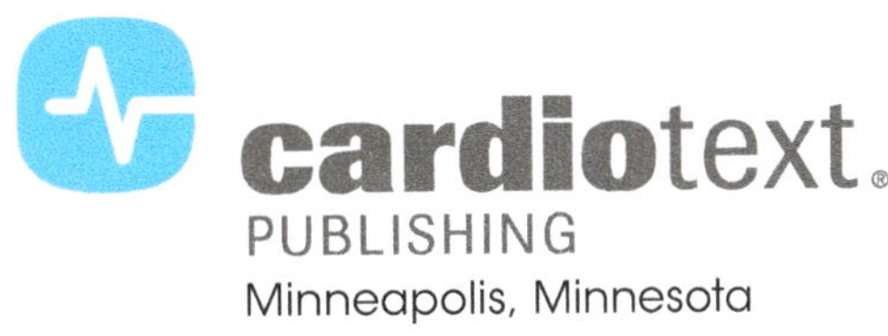

cardiotext.
PUBLISHING
Minneapolis, Minnesota

Cardiotext Publishing, LLC
3405 W. 44th Street
Minneapolis, Minnesota 55410
USA

www.cardiotextpublishing.com

Any updates to this book may be found at: www.cardiotextpublishing.com/electrophysiology-heart-rhythm-mgmt
/the-origins-of-ventricular-arrhythmias

Comments, inquiries, and requests for bulk sales can be directed to the publisher at: info@cardiotextpublishing.com.

Library of Congress Control Number: 2018939965

ISBN: 978-1-942909-22-4

eISBN: 978-1-942909-27-9

Printed in the United States of America

2 3 4 5 6 7   22 21 20 19

To Claire, Max, and Lulu.

Ventricular arrhythmias remain a challenge for the clinical electrophysiologist. But, thanks to Frank Bogun, MD, an internationally recognized expert in this field, *The Origins of Ventricular Arrhythmias: Using the ECG as a Key Tool for Localization* is a valuable addition to every electrophysiology library. This casebook shines a spotlight on the electrocardiography, localization, and mapping of ventricular arrhythmias. This subject is not covered well anywhere else. The cases feature a clinical history, followed by a question, and then the answer is shown with mapping and ablation data as well as up-to-date references. Likewise, the maps and ECGs are superb.

I believe this book is an excellent aid for board preparation. The cases are a great resource and test one's approach to ventricular arrhythmias for localization and ablation.

We are grateful to Frank Bogun for sharing his expertise with mapping and ablation of ventricular arrhythmias with us.

Kenneth A. Ellenbogen, MD
Martha M. and Harold W. Kimmerling Professor of Cardiology
Virginia Commonwealth University School of Medicine
Richmond, Virginia

This book originated from a series of patients who underwent ablation procedures for ventricular arrhythmias at the University of Michigan over the past 2 years. The fellows involved in the cases selected the main arrhythmia and sent the 12-lead ECG, as well as any other pertinent tracings to other fellows in the form of an unknown arrhythmia. Every fellow subsequently submitted a response localizing the origin of the arrhythmia with an appropriate explanation to me. At the end of the week, based on the responses, I sent the fellows the actual site of origin of the arrhythmia, as well as some hints on how to localize the site of origin. These cases demonstrate that previously reported localization criteria often cannot be easily applied, and for some of the cases, such as those with an intramural origin, definite criteria remain to be determined. Our fellows enjoyed solving these ECG riddles; my hope is that this book will be helpful for other electrophysiology and general cardiology fellows to improve their understanding of the 12-lead ECG as a key localizing tool for ventricular arrhythmias.

> This book presents the cases as a series of "unknowns." For the reader interested in reviewing a specific type of case, or the answers to the questions, please note that there is an appendix provided at the end of the book that identifies the origin of the VT or PVC.

AIV	anterior interventricular vein
AL	anterolateral
ARVC/D	arrhythmogenic right ventricular cardiomyopathy/dysplasia
BBRVT	bundle branch reentry VT
CVS	coronary venous system
EAM	electroanatomic map
GCV	great cardiac vein
HPS	His-Purkinje fiber system
IA	inferior axis
ICD	implantable cardioverter-defibrillator
LAD	left anterior descending
LBBB	left bundle branch block
LBBBIA	left bundle branch block inferior axis
LCC	left coronary cusp
LV	left ventricle/left ventricular
LVOT	left ventricular outflow tract
MVA	mitral valve annulus
NYHA	New York Heart Association
PA	pulmonary artery
PAP	papillary muscle
PM	posteromedial
PV	perforator vein
PVC	premature ventricular complex
RBBB	right bundle branch block
RCC	right coronary cusp
RF	radiofrequency
RV	right ventricle/right ventricular
RVOT	right ventricular outflow tract
SA	superior axis
SOO	site of origin
TVA	tricuspid valve annulus
VT	ventricular tachycardia

GLOSSARY

Pace mapping: Pacing from the catheter tip of the mapping catheter aiming to replicate the morphology of a targeted ventricular arrhythmia. For reentrant VTs, a matching pace map indicates an exit site and for idiopathic VAs or focal arrhythmias, it indicates the site of origin.

CLINICAL HISTORY

A 47-year-old man presented with recurrent palpitations and decreased left ventricular ejection fraction of 45%. He had frequent premature ventricular complexes (PVC) with a PVC burden of 24% based on a Holter monitor. He had no delayed enhancement on cardiac MRI and no ischemia on stress testing. Beta-blocker therapy failed to reduce his palpitations. The patient was agreeable to an ablation procedure.

Question

Figure 1.1 shows the 12-lead ECG of the predominant PVC. Where does the PVC originate?

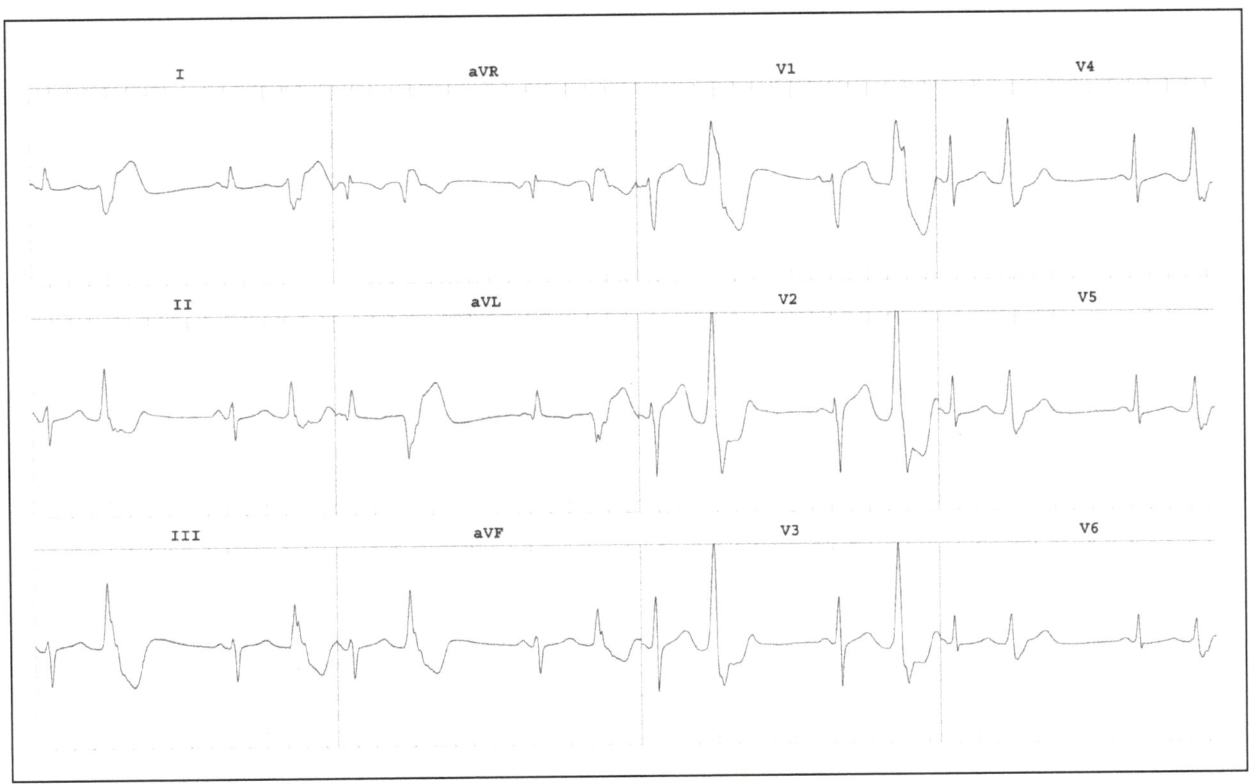

Figure 1.1 A 12-lead ECG showing a bigeminal rhythm with right bundle branch block inferior axis (RBBBIA) morphology.

Answer

The origin of the PVC was the lateral mitral valve annulus (MVA). This needs to be distinguished from an origin at the anterolateral (AL) papillary muscle (PAP). In fact, the pace map from the PAP was very similar to the pace map from the site of origin (SOO) at the MVA. The R/S transition here is lead V_6. Usually for PAP arrhythmias, the transition is earlier, at V_4 or sometimes V_3, but it can also be at V_5 or V_6.[1] Tada et al.[2] describe s and S waves in leads V_6, but at the time of their publication in 2005, PAP arrhythmias had not yet been described as a distinct entity, and some of their patients might have had PAP arrhythmias. If the transition is at lead V_5/V_6 in patients with PAP arrhythmias, the PAP may insert closer to the MVA. It is even possible that the PAP inserts directly

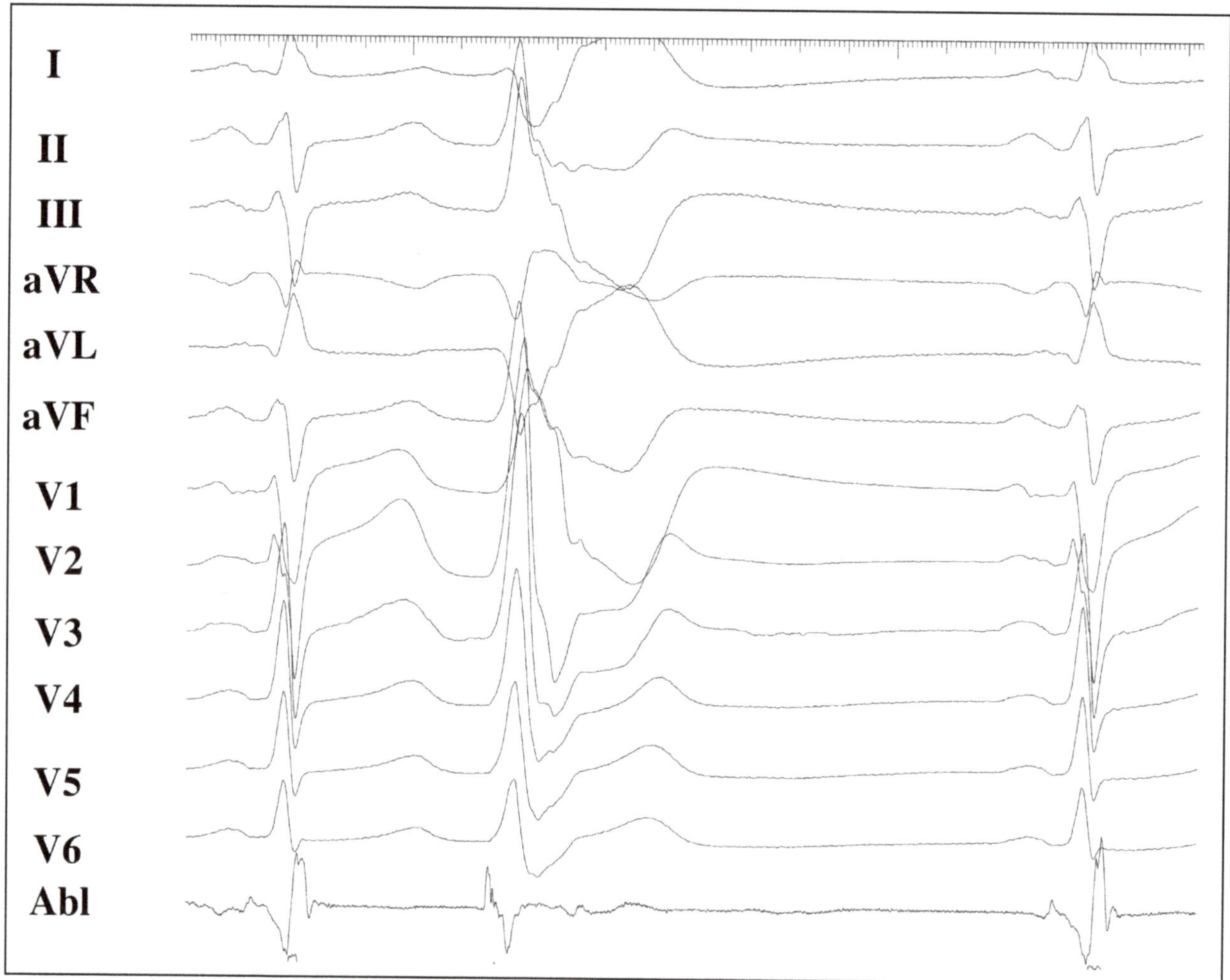

Figure 1.2 Intracardiac tracings from the ablation catheter (Abl) at the site of origin in the anterolateral mitral valve annulus. The local activation time is −25 ms.

into the MVA (this is also called mitral arcade or hammock valve). This results in positive concordance without transition. For arrhythmias originating further away from the anterior MVA, i.e., the lateral or posterior MVA, there is often no positive concordance as one might expect and the transition, despite an annular origin, may be at V_4–V_6. Therefore, PAP origins will need to be kept in the differential for this case as well. At the SOO, the local activation time was –25 ms (**Figure 1.2**) with a matching pace map (**Figure 1.3**) when pacing was performed at this site (**Figure 1.4**). A matching pace map at a site of early activation indicates that the catheter is located at or close to the SOO of the ventricular arrhythmia. If the pace map does not match at a site with early activation, the origin may be located deeper in the tissue.

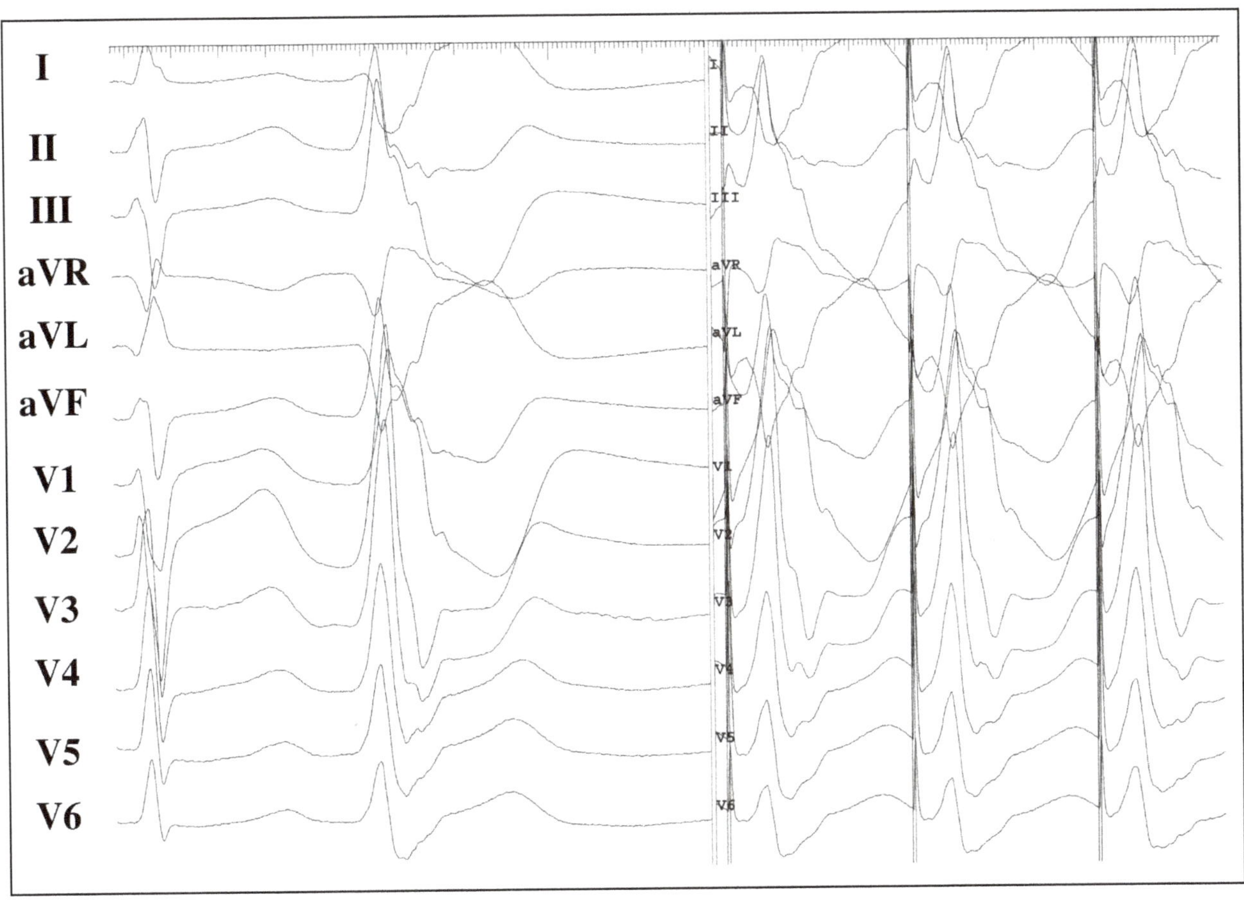

Figure 1.3   **Left panel:** A 12-lead ECG of the targeted PVC. **Right panel:** Pace mapping at the site of origin indicating a match of the pace map with the targeted PVC morphology.

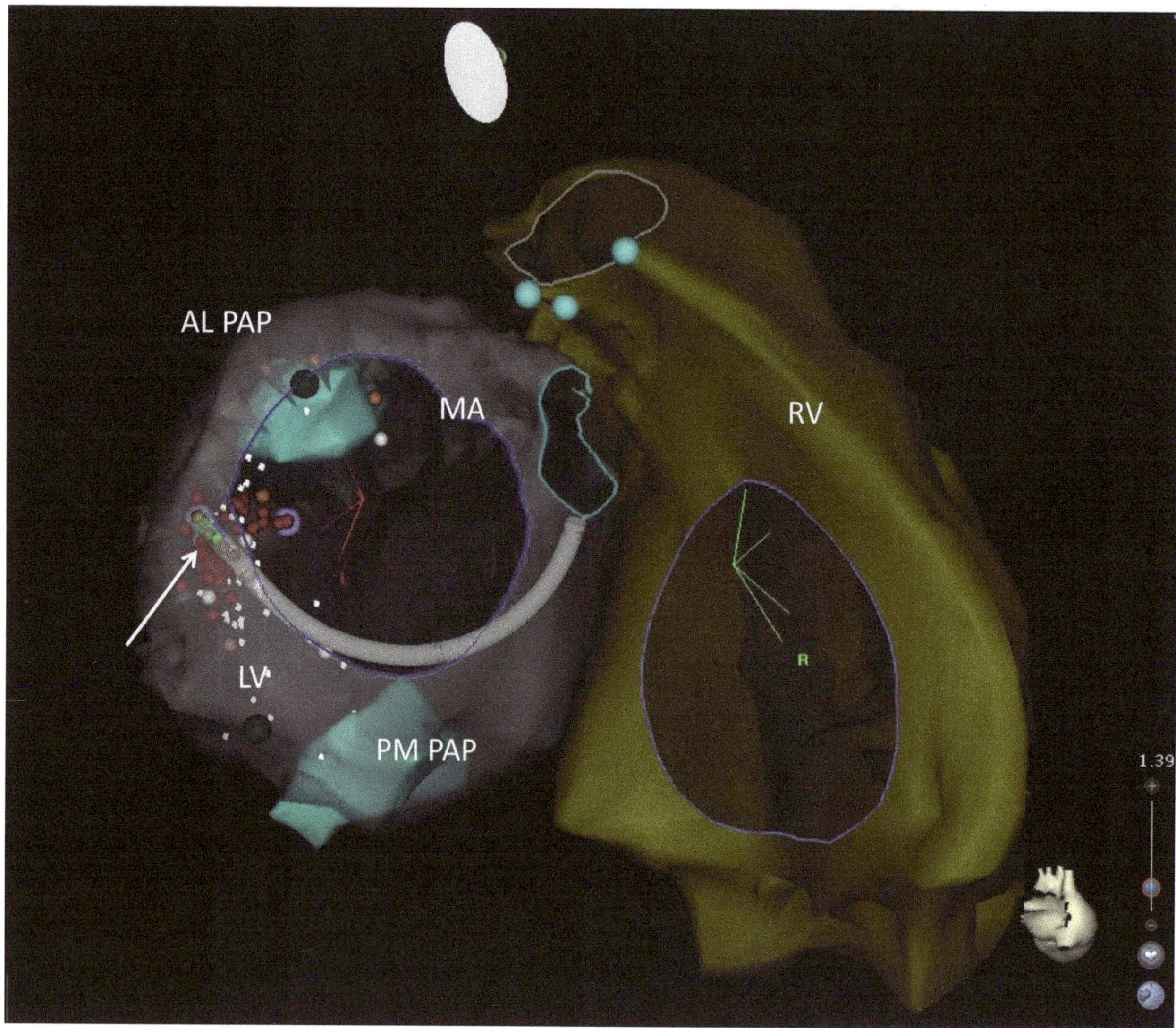

Figure 1.4 A posterior view of the 3D reconstruction of the intracardiac echocardiographic contours of left and right ventricles (RV and LV). The catheter is shown with the tip at the site of origin at the anterolateral mitral valve annulus (**white arrow**). **Red tags** indicate the sites where radiofrequency energy was delivered. The papillary muscles are also displayed in green with the anterolateral papillary muscle (AL PAP) located at 11 o'clock and the posteromedial papillary muscle (PM PAP), located at a 6 o'clock position of the mitral annulus (MA).

REFERENCES

1. Good E, Desjardins B, Jongnarangsin K, et al. Ventricular arrhythmias originating from a papillary muscle in patients without prior infarction: A comparison with fascicular arrhythmias. *Heart Rhythm.* 2008;5:1530–1537.
2. Tada H, Ito S, Naito S, et al. Idiopathic ventricular arrhythmia arising from the mitral annulus: A distinct subgroup of idiopathic ventricular arrhythmias. *J Am Coll Cardiol.* 2005;45:877–886.

CLINICAL HISTORY

A 58-year-old man presented with nonischemic cardiomyopathy and an ejection fraction of 32%. Based on imaging, there was a lateral left wall scar noted on the MRI. He had frequent PVCs, with a PVC burden of 35%, and presented for PVC ablation after an attempted ablation procedure elsewhere failed. A total of seven different PVCs were present; attached is one of his clinical PVCs.

Question

Where does the PVC shown in **Figure 2.1** originate from?

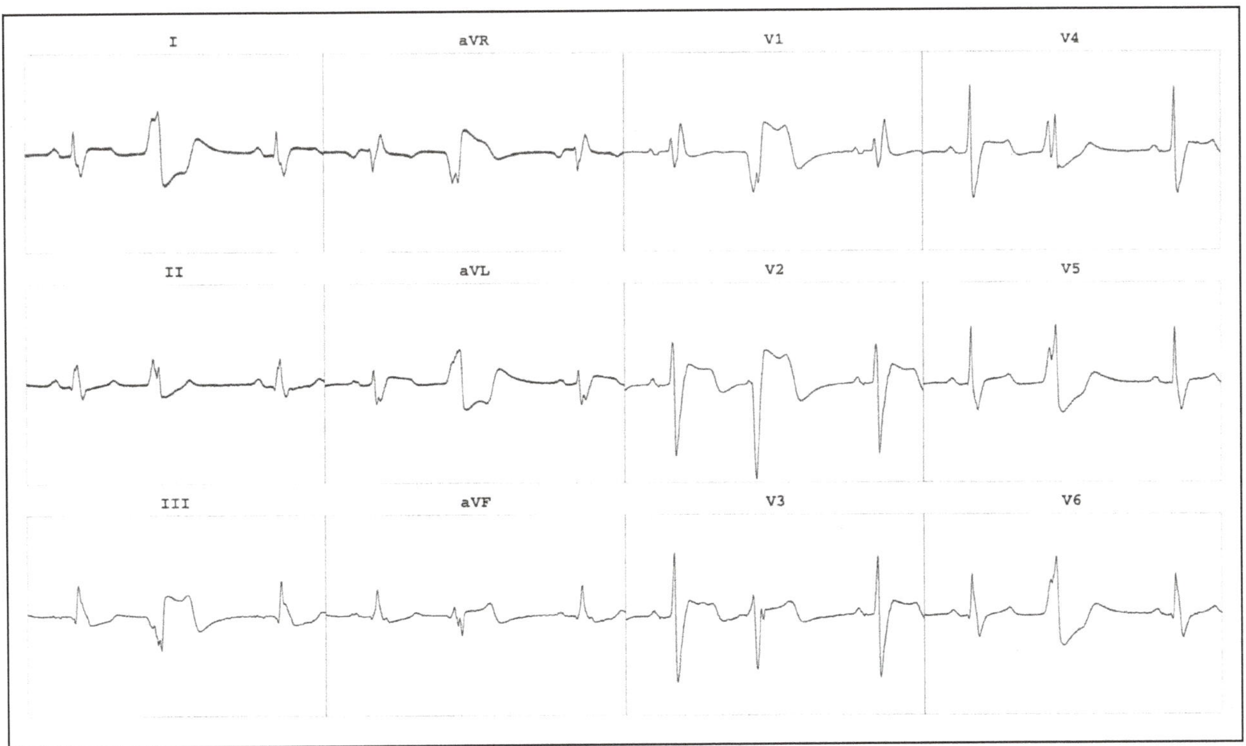

Figure 2.1   A 12-lead ECG of the patient's PVC.

Answer

The PVC originates from the posteroseptal tricuspid valve area close to the bundle of His. The features suggestive of an origin close to the His bundle are: Q wave in lead V_1, R-wave amplitude in lead I > R-wave amplitude of the inferior leads, initial R wave in lead aVL. This constellation should prompt the operator to start the mapping procedure in the tricuspid valve area, close to the His area.[1] The ECG is not precise enough to indicate how close the SOO is located to the His. In this case, the origin was about 1 cm distal to the maximal His bundle deflection on the inferior wall and could be ablated from there at a site with an activation time of −27 ms (**Figure 2.2**) and a matching pace map (**Figure 2.3**). The R wave in lead I is larger than for right ventricular outflow tract (RVOT) arrhythmias because the parahisian/tricuspid valve area is located more to the right side of the RVOT (**Figure 2.4**). This is also the reason for a positive initial deflection in aVL. Often the R-wave transition in the precordial leads is much earlier at V_2/V_3 and not at V_4 as in this case.

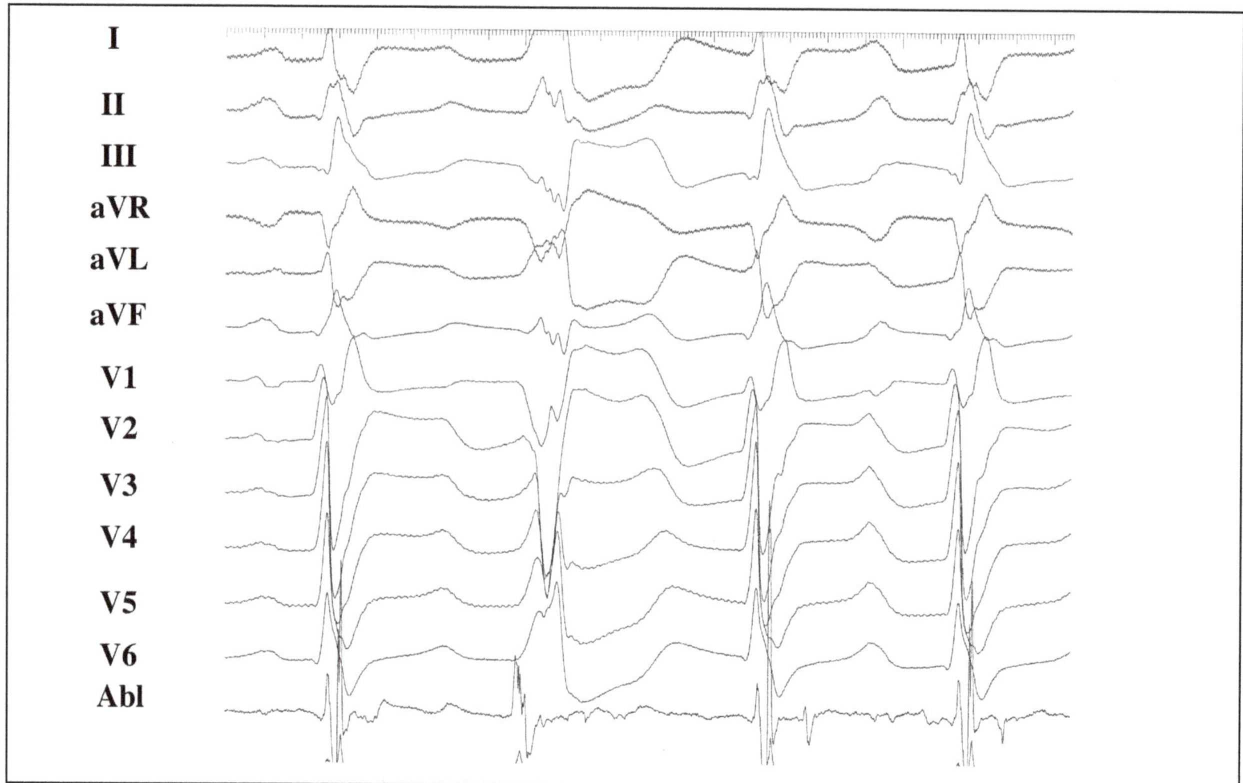

Figure 2.2 Intracardiac electrogram of the site of origin of the PVC. The local activation time was −22 ms.

The later the R-wave transition, the more likely it is that the origin is on the lateral free wall. There is a discrepancy between the inferior leads II and III, since they are not all positive or negative. This is often the case for arrhythmias originating from the level of the tricuspid valve annulus (TVA).[2] The fact that lead II is greater than lead III argues for a more right-sided origin (as compared to the high RVOT, which is located more leftward compared to the low RVOT, Figure 2.4); this observation is not that helpful because the amplitude in the inferior leads is too low (or even negative in lead III), suggesting that the origin is not from the high RVOT. In the higher RVOT, if all inferior leads are positive, an amplitude of II > III would indicate that the origin is more from the right RVOT, i.e., the posterior part of the RVOT; if III > II, it would indicate an origin that is further to the left part of the RVOT, i.e., more superior and possibly from the pulmonary artery (PA).

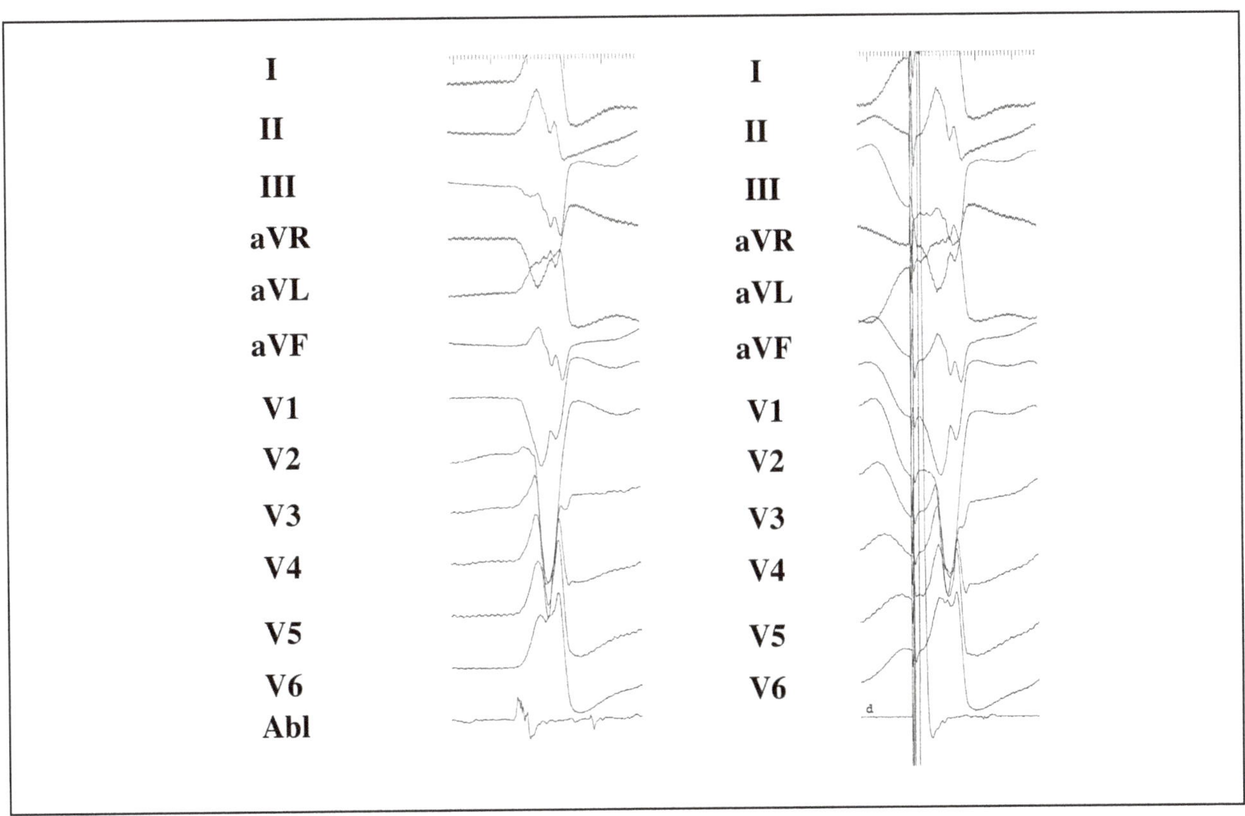

Figure 2.3 **Left panel:** The 12-lead morphology of the targeted PVC. **Right panel:** The morphology of the pace map at the site of origin. There is a matching pace map indicating that the site of origin is located in the endocardium, as opposed to deeper in the tissue.

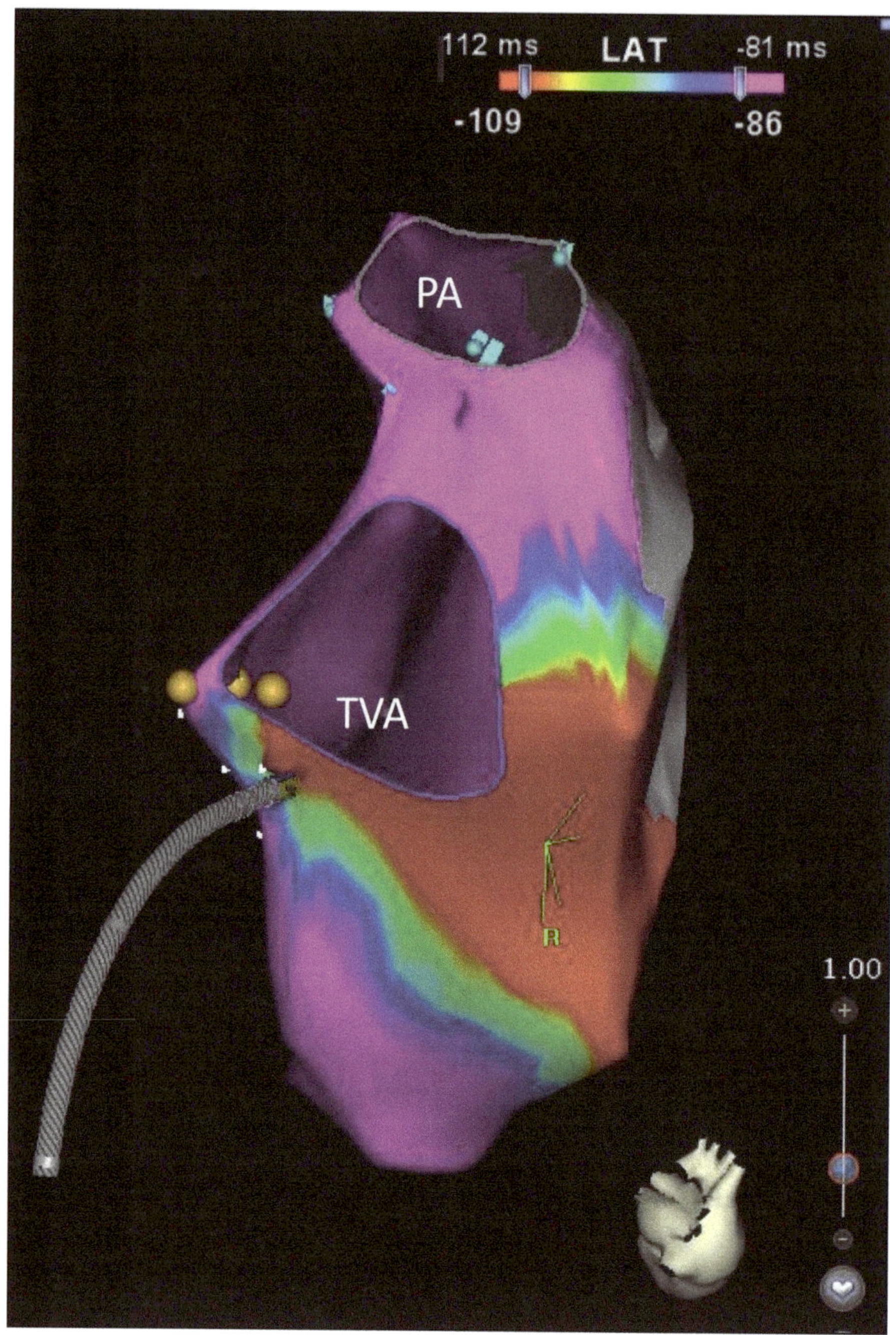

Figure 2.4 Activation map of a posterior view of the right ventricle and the tricuspid valve. The catheter is shown with the tip at the site of origin at the tricuspid valve annulus (TVA). **Red tags** indicate the sites where radiofrequency energy was delivered. The pulmonary artery (PA) is indicated. The location of the His bundle is indicated with orange tags.

REFERENCES

1. Yamauchi Y, Aonuma K, Takahashi A, et al. Electrocardiographic characteristics of repetitive monomorphic right ventricular tachycardia originating near the His-bundle. *J Cardiovasc Electrophysiol*. 2005;16:1041–1048.
2. Tada H, Tadokoro K, Ito S, et al. Idiopathic ventricular arrhythmias originating from the tricuspid annulus: Prevalence, electrocardiographic characteristics, and results of radiofrequency catheter ablation. *Heart Rhythm*. 2007;4:7–16.

CLINICAL HISTORY

A 76-year-old man with a history of aortic valve replacement and nonischemic cardiomyopathy with an ejection fraction ranging from 20%–45%. His PVC burden was 40%. There was no scar in the cardiac MRI.

Question

Where does the PVC shown in **Figure 3.1** originate, and what is the differential diagnosis regarding the origin of the PVC?

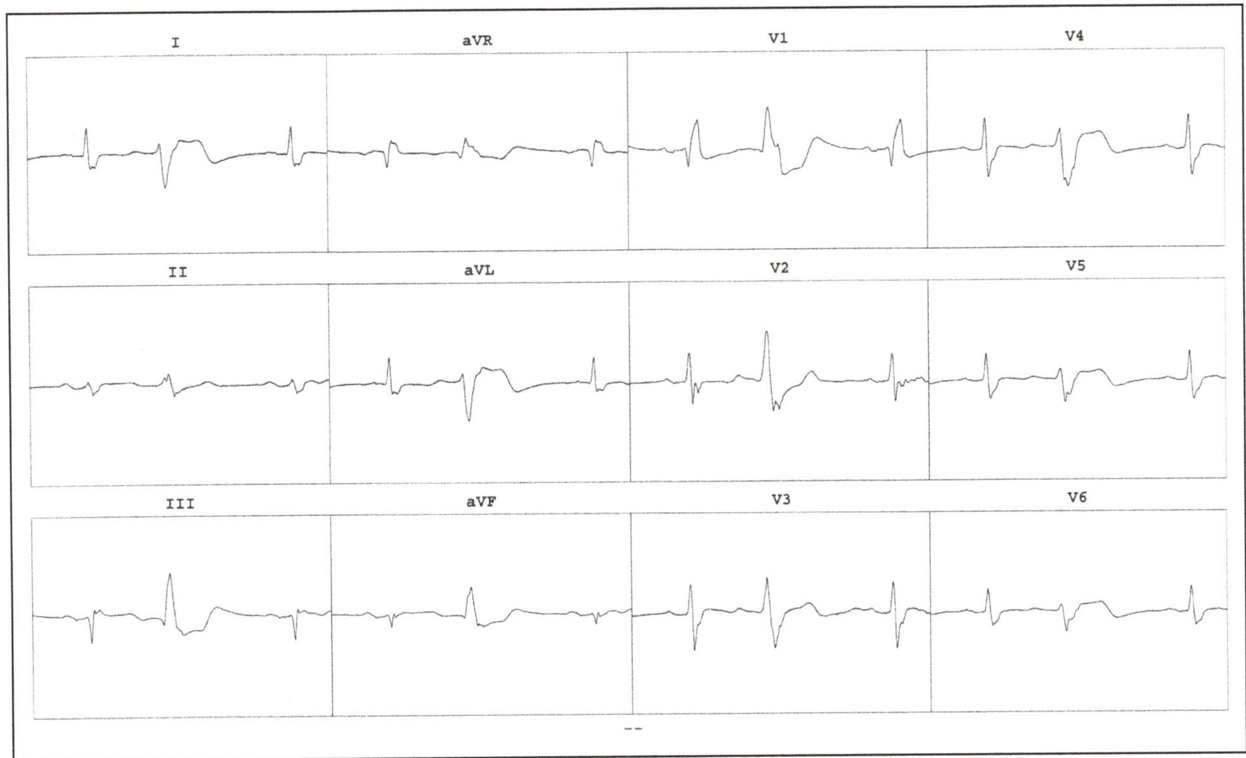

Figure 3.1   A 12-lead ECG of the patient's PVC.

Answer

The origin of the PVC is the anterolateral papillary muscle (**Figure 3.2**). It has a right bundle branch block (RBBB) right axis morphology with a transition in lead V_3/V_4. The differential is a fascicular origin and an origin at the mitral annulus. Distinguishing features include: QRS width: > 120–140 ms, lack of rsR′ in V_1 for fascicular origin, and the lack of positive concordance for a mitral valve origin.[1,2] Given the broader QRS morphology, the origin is likely to be from the PAP. The rightward axis indicates an origin from the anterolateral PAP; a leftward axis would indicate an origin from the posteromedial PAP. The late transition also favors an origin from the PAP as opposed to the mitral annulus, where one would expect to see a positive concordance in the precordial leads.

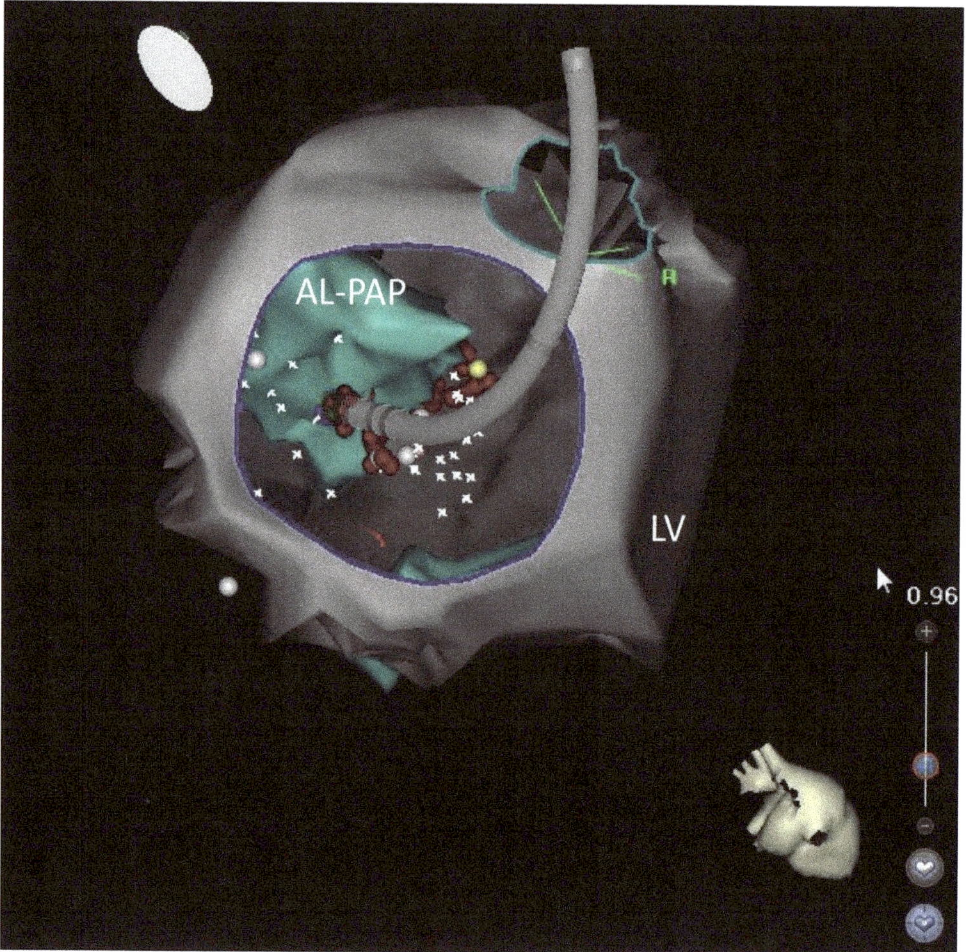

Figure 3.2 A 3D reconstruction of the echocardiographic shell of the left ventricle (LV) and the anterolateral papillary muscle (AL PAP **colored in green**). The catheter is positioned at a site that was critical for the PVC shown in Figure 3.1.

REFERENCES

1. Good E, Desjardins B, Jongnarangsin K, et al. Ventricular arrhythmias originating from a papillary muscle in patients without prior infarction: A comparison with fascicular arrhythmias. *Heart Rhythm*. 2008;5:1530–1537.
2. Al'Aref SJ, Ip JE, Markowitz SM, et al. Differentiation of papillary muscle from fascicular and mitral annular ventricular arrhythmias in patients with and without structural heart disease. *Circ Arrhythm Electrophysiol*. 2015;8:616–624.

CLINICAL HISTORY

A 67-year-old woman was admitted to the emergency department (ED) with palpitations and dizziness. She had intermittent palpitations over the past 6 months. Initially, they occurred once a month, but increased over the past month to occur on a daily basis and last up to a minute. Symptoms include lightheadedness. She had one episode of syncope a few months ago. In the ED, she had multiple episodes of documented regular, wide complex tachycardia with a rate of 188 bpm lasting up to 40 seconds and terminating spontaneously. On an ECG, she had preserved left ventricular function; cardiac catheterization was normal.

Question

Where does the arrhythmia shown in **Figure 4.1** originate?

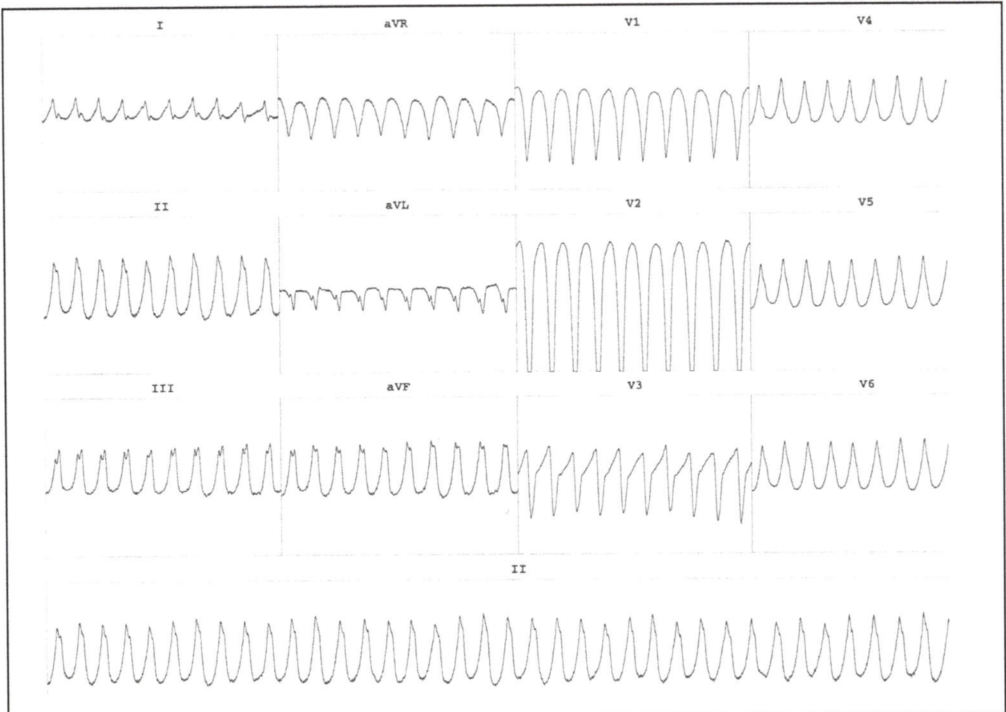

Figure 4.1   A 12-lead ECG of the induced clinical VT.

The arrhythmia is a rapid ventricular tachycardia (VT) with a cycle length of 260 ms. The VT originated from the anterior aspect of the RVOT just below the pulmonic valve. There was surprisingly a large amount of low voltage in that region. The localization based on the 12-lead morphology would have predicted a posterior origin; i.e., positive QRS in lead I and amplitude of lead II > lead III because the anterior RVOT is oriented more leftward compared to the posterior RVOT, which is more rightward-oriented (i.e., lead I is positive and lead II > lead III).[1] In the current case, the scar may have contributed to the different morphology, i.e., by routing the activation more

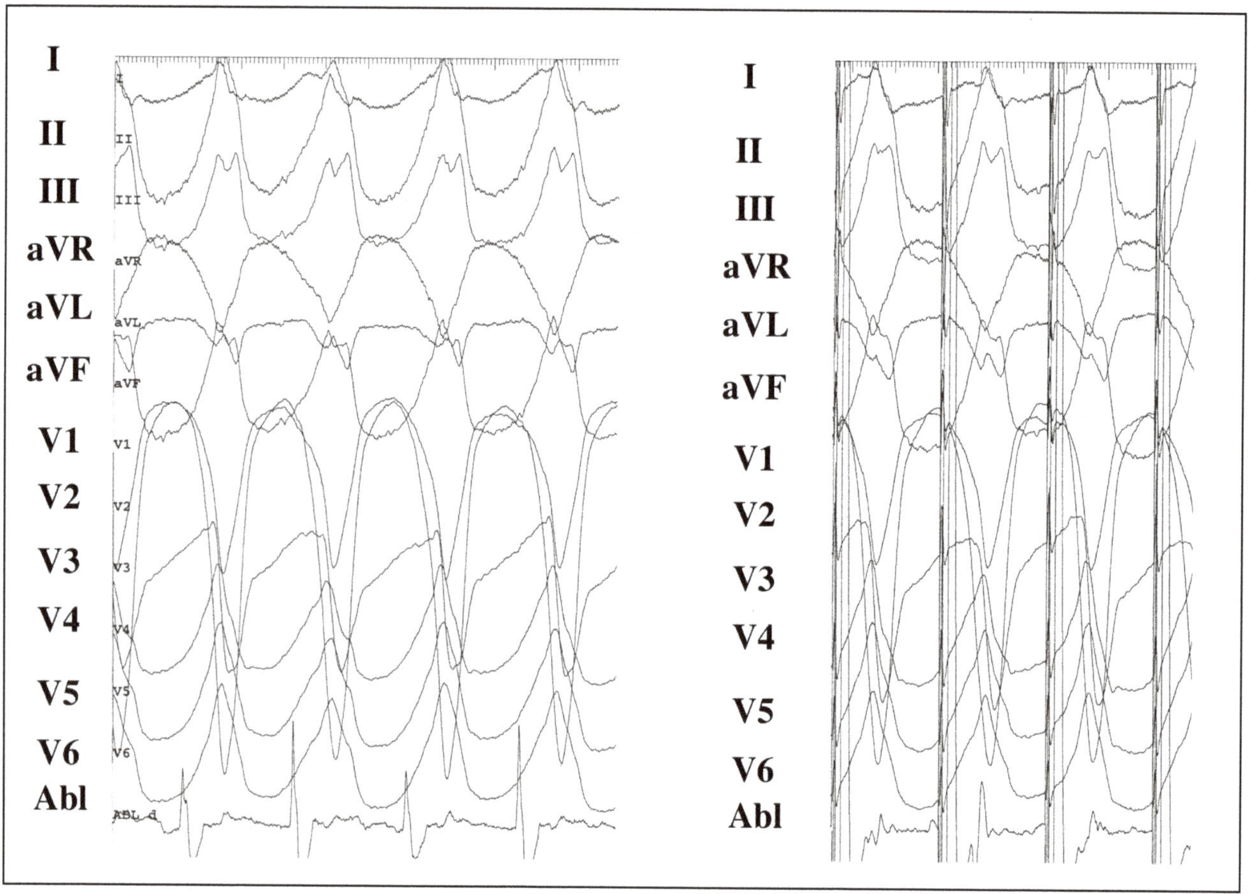

Figure 4.2 **Left panel:** The site of origin is indicated and the activation time was −30 ms. **Right panel:** Pace mapping the anterior region of the RVOT below the pulmonic valve showed a large area of matching pace maps.

posteriorly than anteriorly. The late transition and the notching further indicate that the VT originates from the RV free wall as opposed to the septum.

Lead aVL is not particularly helpful for distinction of the origin within the high RVOT. Lead aVL is usually negative, indicating that the activation comes from high up in the RVOT. Since the RVOT is mostly located to the left of the RV, the vector goes rightward. The VT was ablated at a site with early timing (–25 ms) where there was a closely matched pace map (**Figure 4.2**) in the anterior RVOT (**Figure 4.3**). The VT was reproducibly inducible prior to the ablation and was no longer inducible after the ablation.

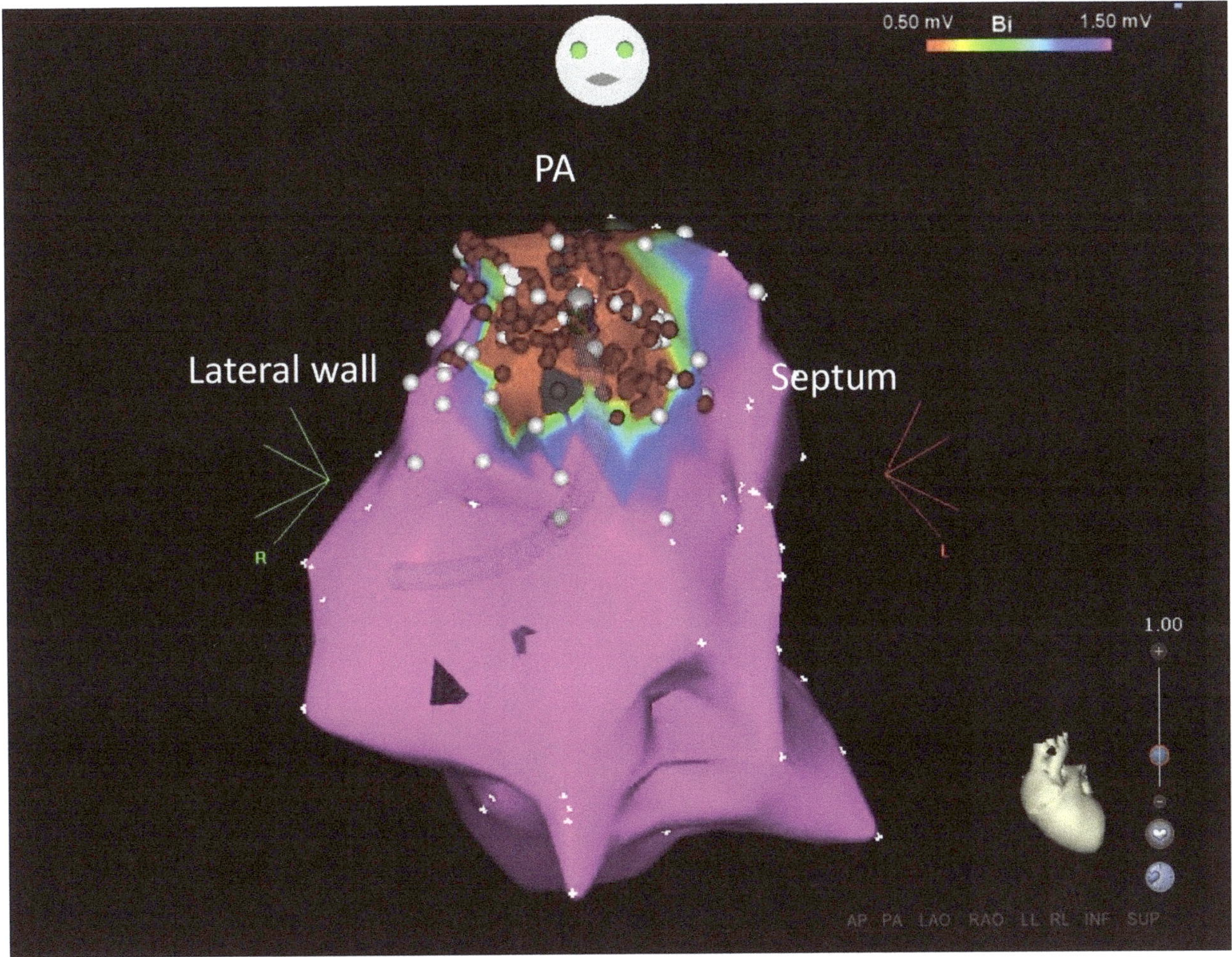

Figure 4.3   This figure shows an electroanatomic bipolar voltage map of the RVOT. There is a large rim of lower, bipolar voltage in the anterior RVOT where the VT originates. The lateral wall, the septum, and the pulmonic valve are indicated. The catheter is at a site with a matching pace map where radiofrequency ablation was performed.

REFERENCE

1. Dixit S, Gerstenfeld EP, Callans DJ, Marchlinski FE. Electrocardiographic patterns of superior right ventricular outflow tract tachycardias: distinguishing septal and free-wall sites of origin. *J Cardiovasc Electrophysiol.* 2003;14:1–7.

CLINICAL HISTORY

A 67-year-old man presented with nonischemic cardiomyopathy and an ejection fraction of 45%. He had an implanted loop recorder that showed multiple episodes of sustained, wide complex tachycardia controlled with sotalol and verapamil combination therapy. A cardiac MRI showed no delayed enhancement.

Question

Where does the arrhythmia shown in **Figure 5.1** originate? What is the mechanism? What is the ablation strategy?

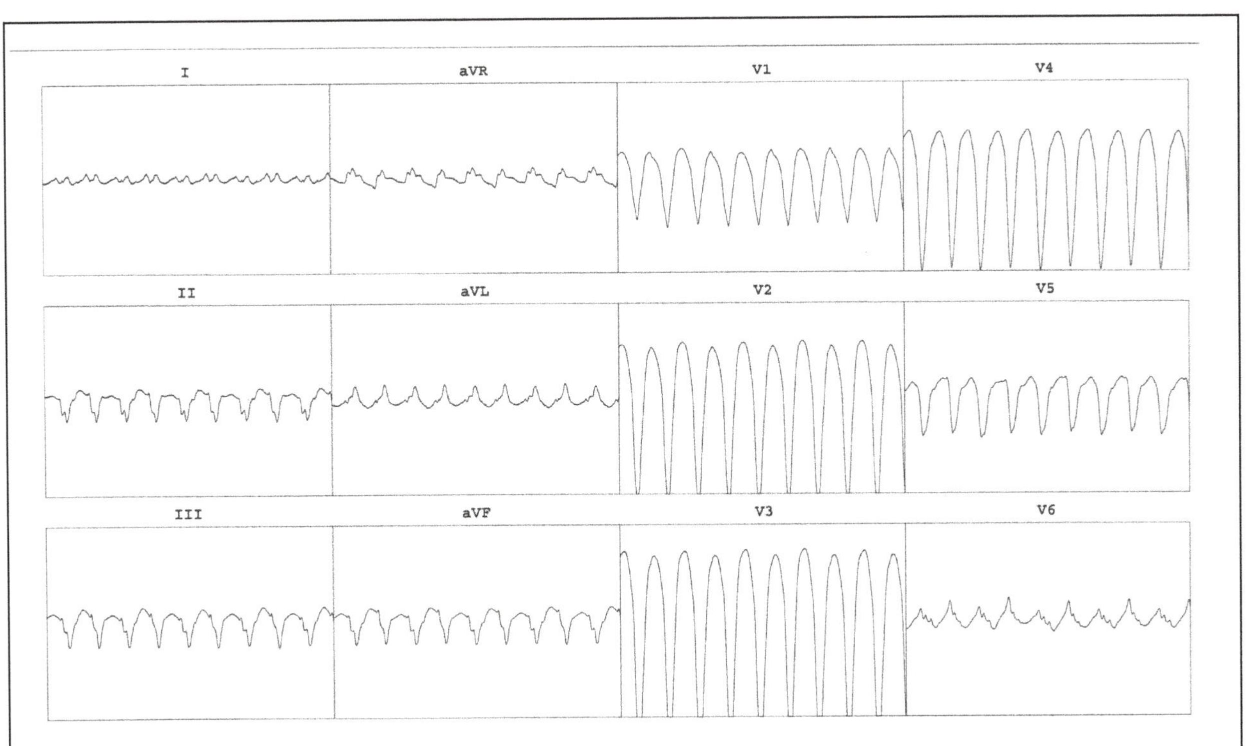

Figure 5.1 A 12-lead ECG showing VT.

The ECG tracings (Figure 5.1) show VT, and specifically bundle branch reentry tachycardia (BBRVT). There is really no perfect clue on this particular ECG to nail down the precise mechanism of this VT. Typical key features for BBRVT are: typical left bundle branch block (LBBB)-QRS morphology, LBBB-QRS morphology identical/similar to the sinus rhythm QRS morphology. The latter was not the case here, because both bundles were equally involved in the disease process, so the QRS complex in sinus rhythm was actually narrow. Other procedural hints were difficult to obtain. For example, there is usually evidence of conduction disease with a long H-V interval. The His bundle could not be identified initially; this is not uncommon in patients in whom the conduction system is diseased, and one has to spend the time required to identify the His bundle potential and demonstrate conduction disease in the His-Purkinje fiber system (HPS). An initial attempt to identify the His bundle failed and was abandoned too quickly, since the His signal was not easily identified. Instead, time was spent on performing activation mapping the inducible VT. Another procedural hint is the postpacing interval obtained from a catheter placed in the RV apex. If within 30 ms, this is also indicative of BBRVT.[1] This important step was also skipped. Instead, pace mapping and then activation mapping were performed in the right ventricular inflow tract.

The superior axis (SA) with the late transition points in the direction of an inferoapical origin of the VT. Matching pace maps (10/12 leads, but no better than that) were found over a large area, including the moderator band. In contrast to VT of myocardial origin, BBRVT with a LBBB pattern characteristically shows rapid deflections in the right precordial leads, indicating that the initial ventricular activation occurs through the HPS—this is really not appreciable in the present case. During BBRVT with a LBBB pattern, the activation runs in the antegrade direction down the right bundle branch and in the retrograde direction up the left bundle branch. During BBRVT with a RBBB pattern, the direction of activation is reversed. The orientation of frontal plane QRS axis is usually to the left. Less frequently, it may be normal or rightward.

An origin from the moderator band is in the differential, and the posterior PAP should be in the differential for the SOO as well. They all have a LBBB morphology, late transition ($\geq V_4$), and may have a rapid deflection (arguing for a proximity closer to the specialized conduction system) with a narrower QRS complex compared to RV free wall origins.[2,3] After delivery of a few radiofrequency (RF) lesions at the moderator band, the VT was still inducible, and we were suspicious about BBRVT, especially since Purkinje potentials were recorded on the moderator band preceding the onset of the QRS complex by 10–15 ms (**Figure 5.2**). Another attempt to localize the His position was made, and the His potential was eventually identified (**Figure 5.3**); it showed an H-V interval

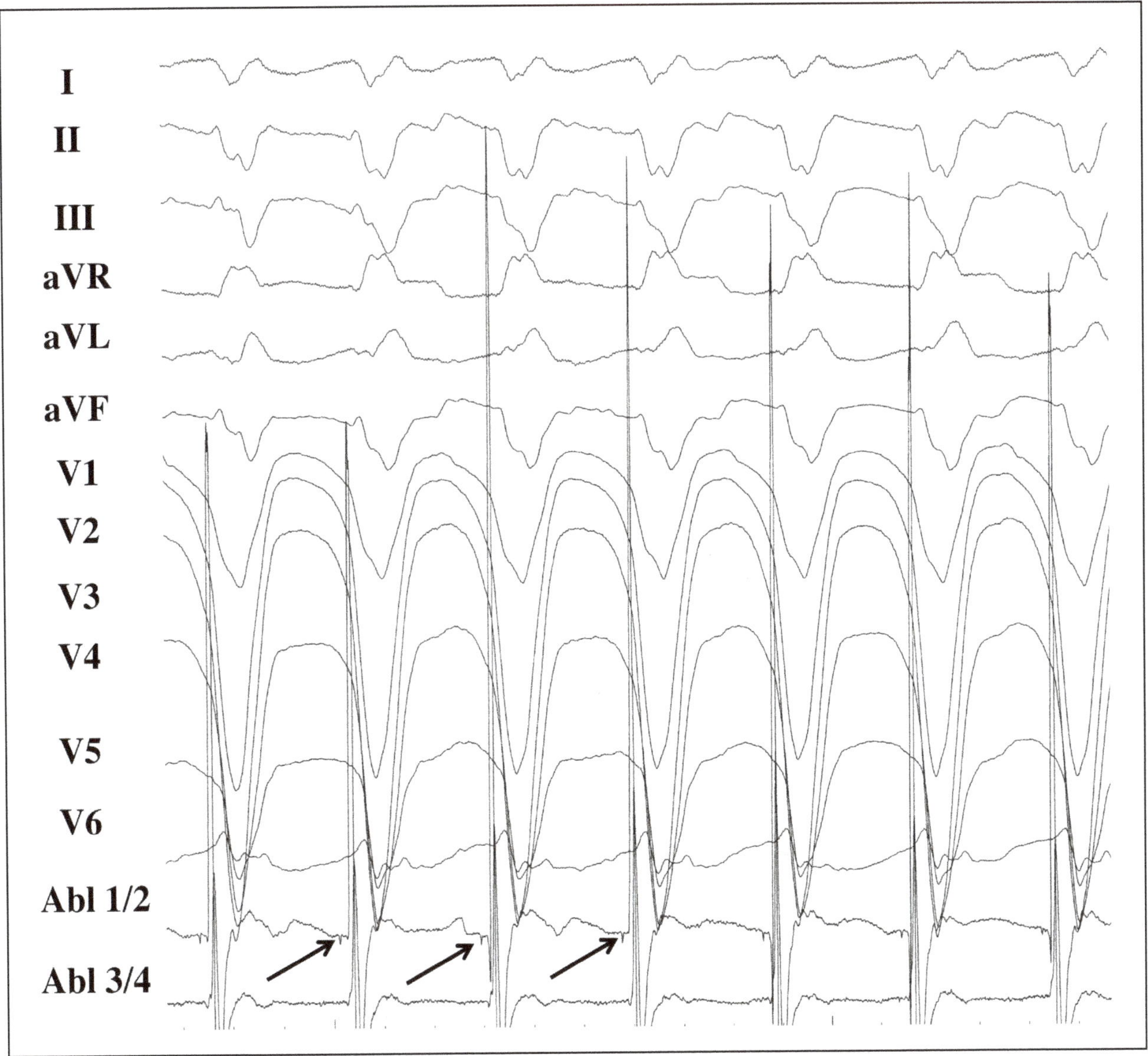

Figure 5.2 A 12-lead ECG with intracardiac recordings from the mapping catheter located at the moderator band. There are Purkinje potentials preceding the QRS by 10 ms (**arrow**).

of 85 ms. The VT was induced with the catheter at the His position and the diagnosis of BBRVT was made based on changes in the R-R interval being preceded by changes in the H-H interval (**Figure 5.4**). The right bundle branch was then identified (**Figure 5.5**) and ablated. Subsequently, the patient was no longer inducible. **Figure 5.6** illustrates the catheter location mapping the moderator band (left panel) and the right bundle branch area (right panel).

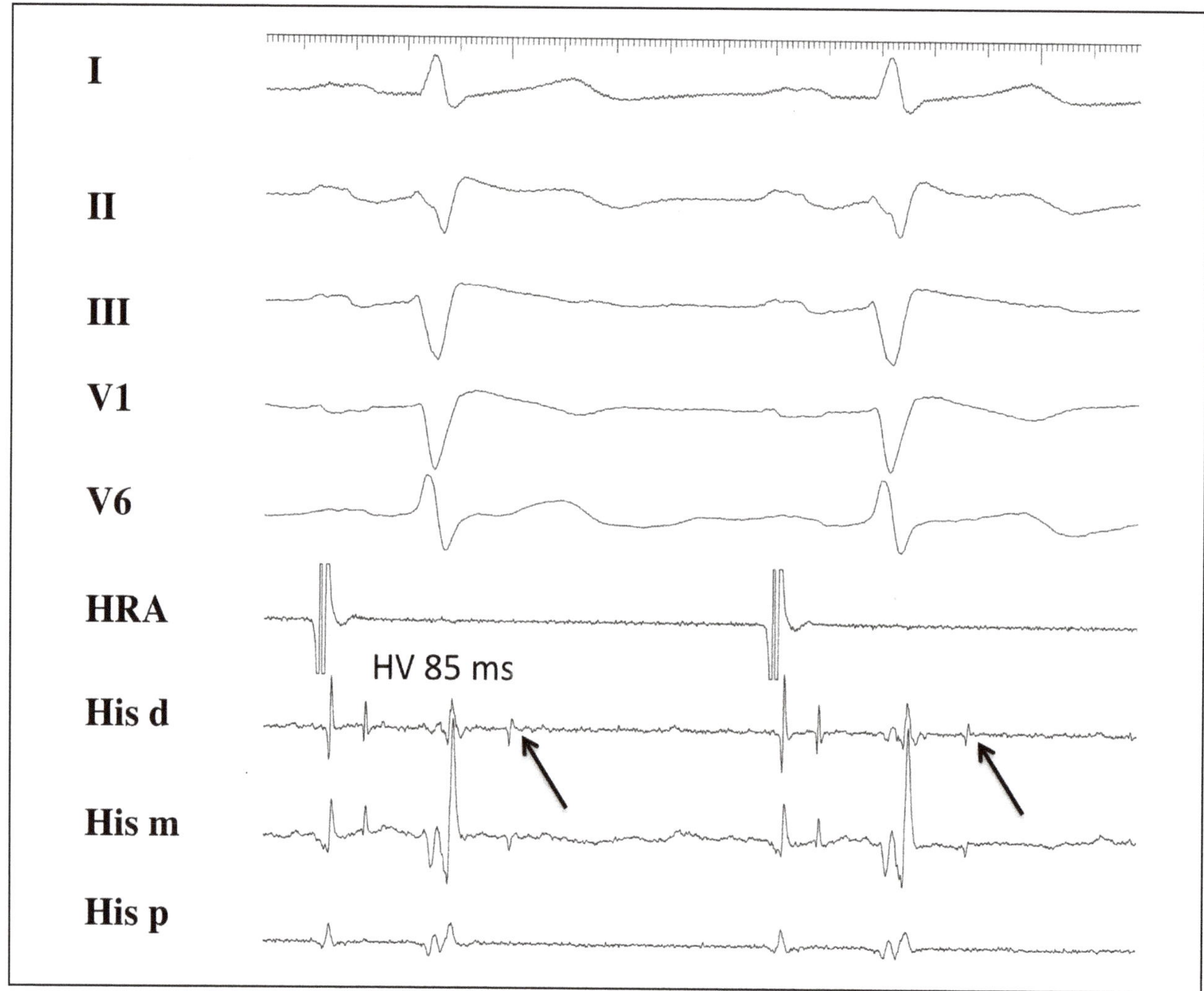

Figure 5.3 Surface ECGs with intracardiac recordings of a catheter in the high right atrium (HRA) and a multipolar catheter at the His bundle position [His distal (d), mid (m), proximal (p)]. The H-V interval measures 85 ms. There are late potentials present (**arrow**), indicating scarring of that region.

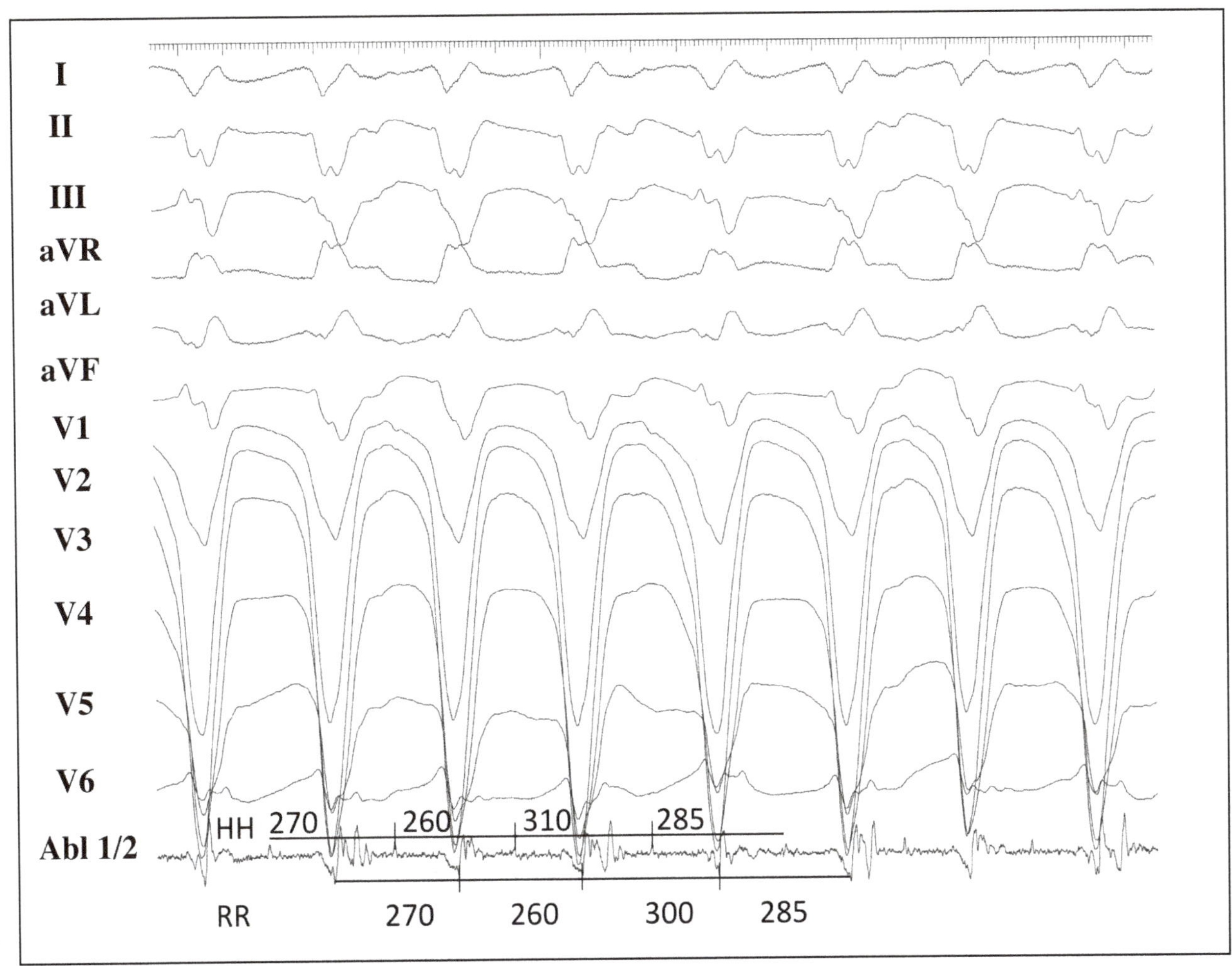

Figure 5.4 A 12-lead ECG obtained during VT with the catheter at the site of the His recording. R-R and V-V intervals are indicated, and changes in the R-R intervals are preceded by changes in the H-H intervals, indicating BBRVT.

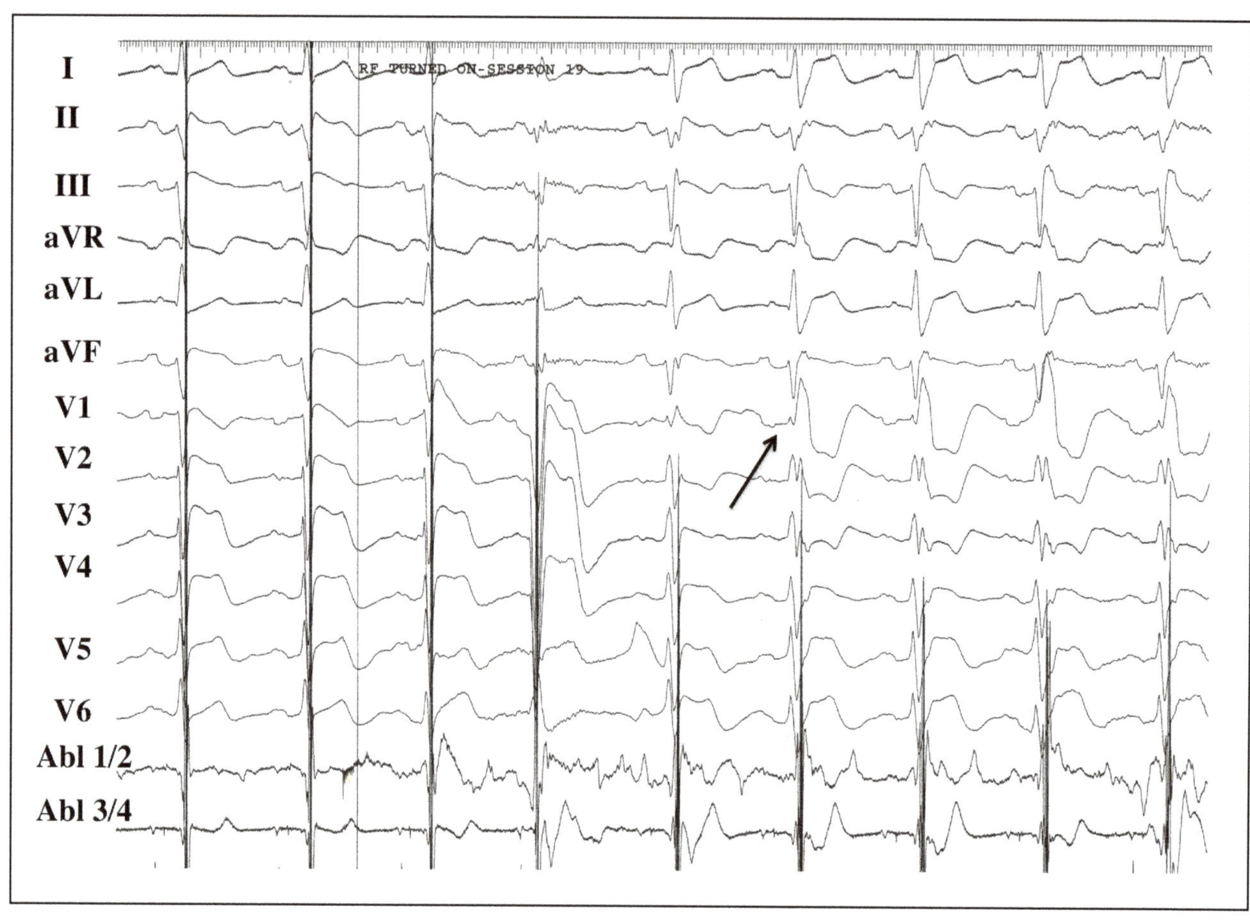

Figure 5.5 An intracardiac tracing of the ablation catheter at a site where the right bundle branch is located and where radiofrequency energy is delivered. This results in a RBBB (**arrow**).

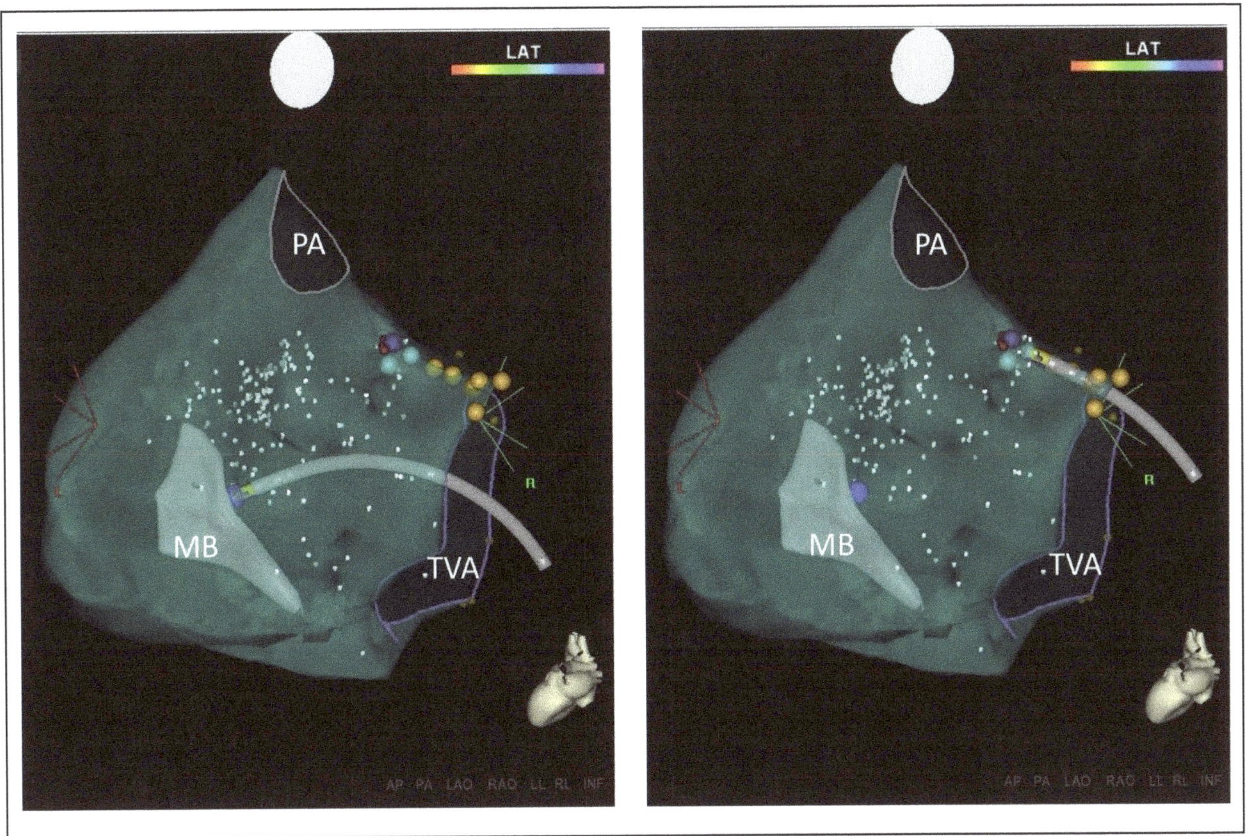

Figure 5.6 This figure shows an anterior view of the 3D reconstruction of the intracardiac echocardiographic contours of right ventricle. The **right panel** shows the catheter in contact with the right bundle branch and the **left panel** shows the ablation catheter in contact with the moderator band (MB) where the right bundle branch inserted. Pulmonic valve (PA) and tricuspid valve annulus (TVA) are also indicated.

REFERENCES

1. Merino JL, Peinado R, Fernandez-Lozano I, Sobrino N, Sobrino JA. Transient entrainment of bundle-branch reentry by atrial and ventricular stimulation: Elucidation of the tachycardia mechanism through analysis of the surface ECG. *Circulation.* 1999;100:1784–1790.
2. Van Herendael H, Garcia F, Lin D, et al. Idiopathic right ventricular arrhythmias not arising from the outflow tract: Prevalence, electrocardiographic characteristics, and outcome of catheter ablation. *Heart Rhythm.* 2011;8:511–518.
3. Sadek MM, Benhayon D, Sureddi R, et al. Idiopathic ventricular arrhythmias originating from the moderator band: Electrocardiographic characteristics and treatment by catheter ablation. *Heart Rhythm.* 2015;12:67–75.

CLINIC HISTORY

A 72-year-old man presented with a history of ischemic cardiomyopathy and two-vessel coronary artery disease involving the right coronary artery and circumflex artery and prior inferolateral myocardial infarction. His ejection fraction was 25%, and he had severe pulmonary hypertension. There was scarring in the inferolateral wall based on the cardiac MRI. The patient was status post-biventricular implanted cardioverter-defibrillator (ICD) implantation, and despite combination of amiodarone and mexelitine, had recurrent ICD therapy for VT. During his ablation procedure, multiple VTs were inducible.

Question

Figure 6.1 shows one of the VTs. Where is this VT originating?

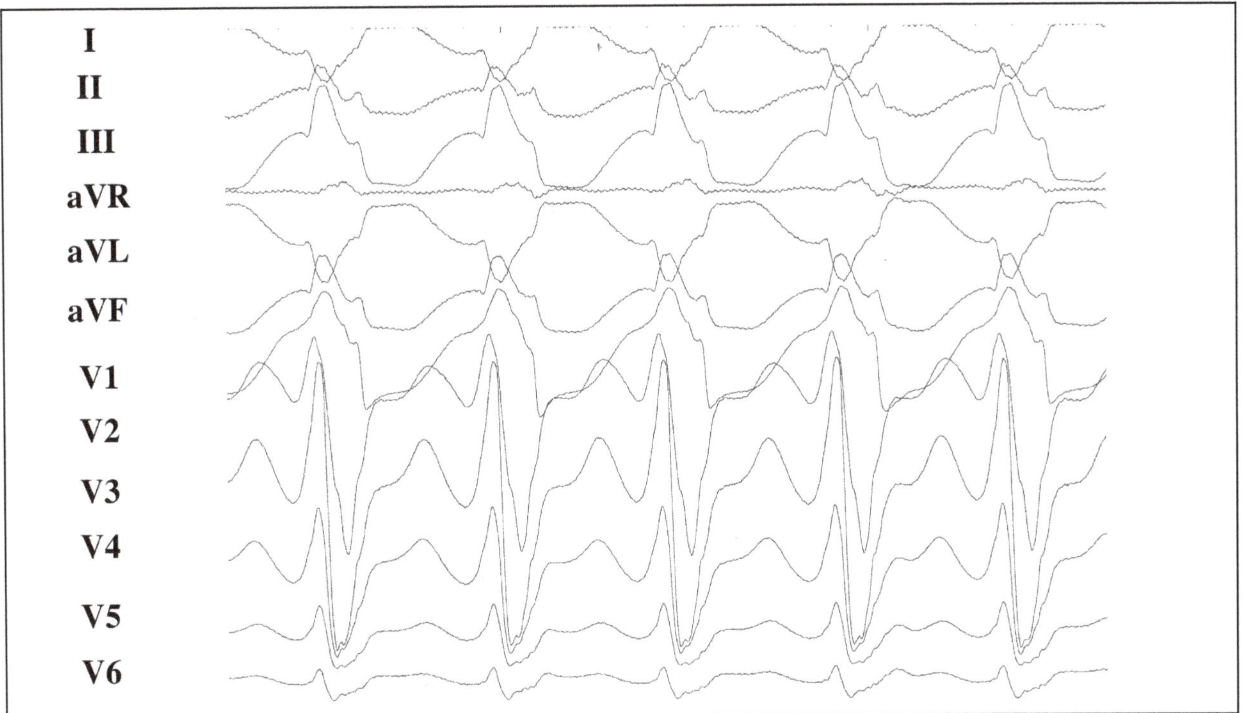

Figure 6.1   A 12-lead ECG of an induced VT.

Answer

The patient's VT originates from the anterior MVA. It is an unusual origin for a patient with an inferior wall myocardial infarction, and this morphology is more often seen in patients with prior anterior wall infarction. However, in this patient the scar extends up to the anterior part of the MVA (**Figure 6.2** and **Figure 6.3**). The anterior PAP muscle would have been another possibility, as the R wave in V_6 that is predominantly positive suggests a more basal origin. A few general remarks about the origin of postinfarction VTs:

- A LBBB morphology in general suggests the origin is from the RV or septum of the LV.

- RBBB morphology in general suggests the origin is from the LV.

- Positive concordance (predominant R waves in all precordial leads): Basal LV origin and predominantly anterior (some can be lateral).

- Negative concordance (i.e., all precordial leads negative): The origin is the apex.

- Q waves usually indicate the myocardial area where the VT is originating (or exiting). In this example, Q waves in II/III/aVF indicate that the exit of the VT is the inferior wall. Q waves in V_1/V_2 indicate that the exit is septal.

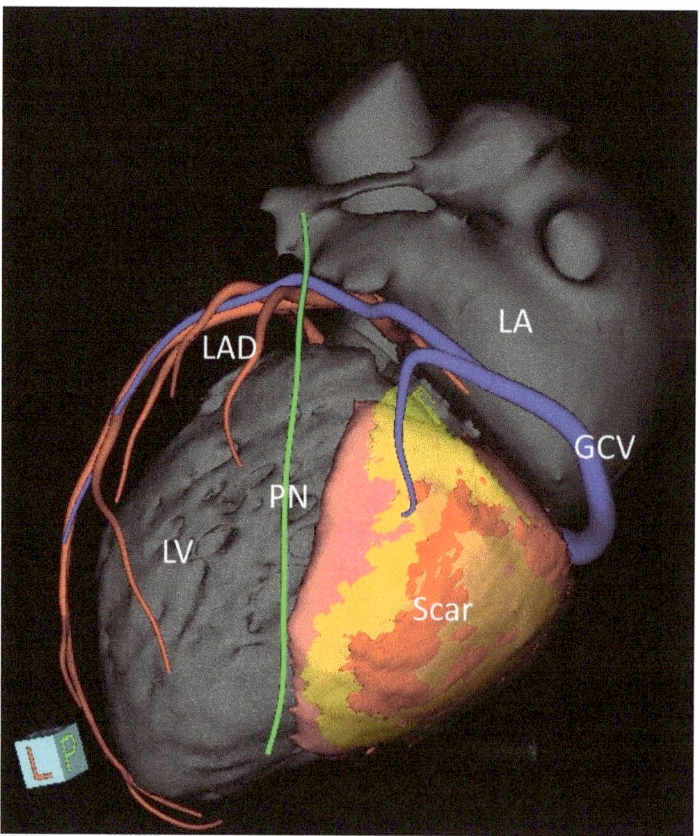

Figure 6.2 A 3D reconstruction of the left lateral ventricular endocardial shell based on cardiac CT and MRI. The coronary arteries (left anterior descending = LAD), the great cardiac vein and the phrenic nerve (PN), and the left atrium (LA) are also shown. There is a large inferolateral scar in the left ventricle (LV).

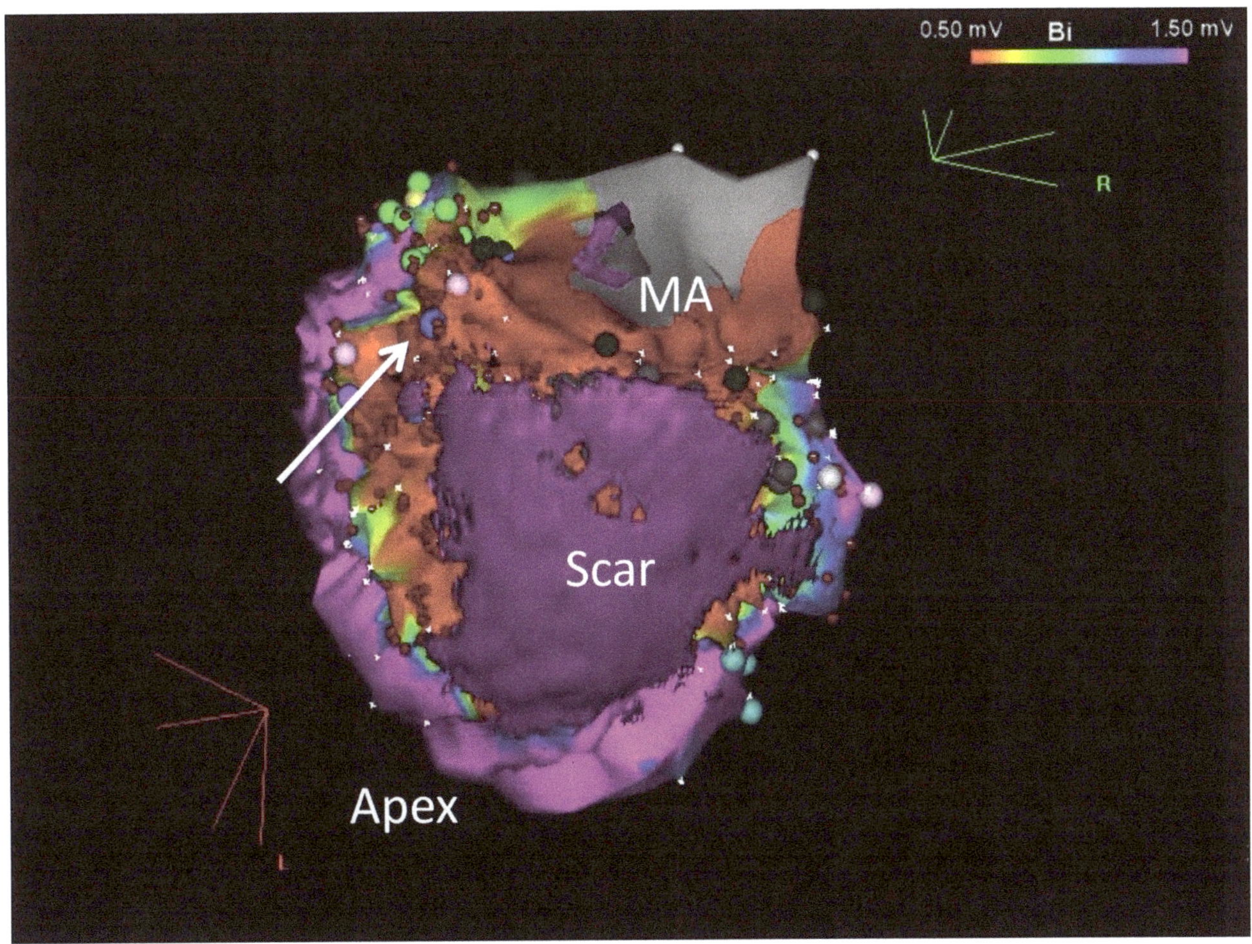

Figure 6.3 This figure shows a bipolar electroanatomical voltage map of the left ventricle viewed from the lateral aspect. The mitral annulus (MA), the left ventricular apex as well as the registered scar from the MRI (**violet**) are indicated. A **blue tag** (**white arrow**) indicates the location where the targeted VT had its exit site.

Using these simple rules, one would correctly localize this arrhythmia to originate from the anterior basal LV. Algorithms indicating the origins of VTs have many limitations,[1] and accuracy of the algorithm described by Miller et al. is only in the ≤ 50% range. A computerized algorithm performed with accuracy in the 70% range.[2]

REFERENCES

1. Miller JM, Marchlinski FE, Buxton AE, Josephson ME. Relationship between the 12-lead electrocardiogram during ventricular tachycardia and endocardial site of origin in patients with coronary artery disease. *Circulation.* 1988;77(4):759–766. PubMed PMID: 3349580.
2. Yokokawa M, Liu TY, Yoshida K, et al. Automated analysis of the 12-lead electrocardiogram to identify the exit site of postinfarction ventricular tachycardia. *Heart Rhythm.* 2012;9(3):330–334. PubMed PMID: 22001707.

CLINICAL HISTORY

A 66-year-old woman presented with VT. She has a history of arrhythmogenic right ventricular cardiomyopathy/dysplasia (ARVC/D) and VT ablation seven years earlier. She was admitted two months ago with VT storm and multiple ICD shocks and was treated with sotalol. Sotalol reduced her VT events. However, she had long, symptomatic episodes of nonsustained VT shown in **Figure 7.1**.

Question

Based on the 12-lead ECG shown in Figure 7.1, where do her arrhythmias originate?

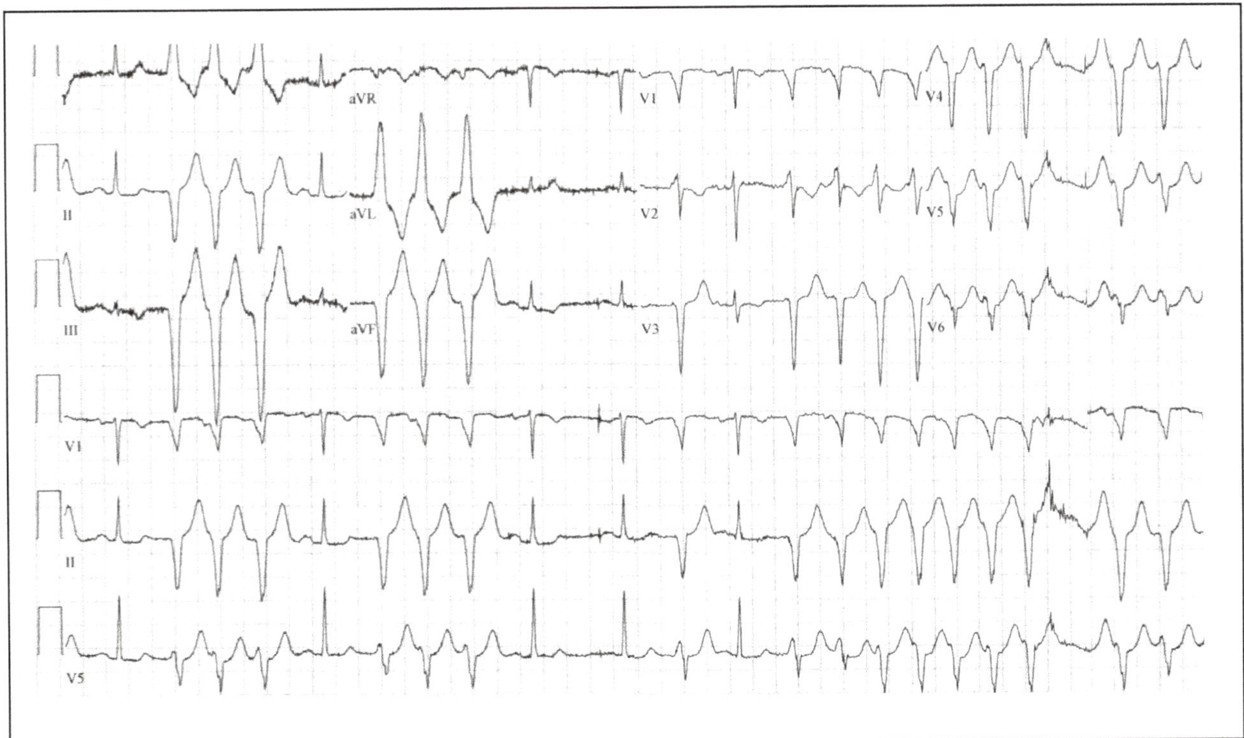

Figure 7.1 A 12-lead ECG with nonsustained VT.

Answer

The origin is the inferior aspect of the tricuspid annulus. However, the ECG pattern is not typical for this location. Most VTs in patients with ARVC/D originate either from the peritricuspid area or the RVOT. One might suspect an epicardial origin based on the well-described "pattern break" in the precordial RV transition seen in V_1–V_3 (i.e., no R wave in V_1, broad R wave in V_2, and decreased or no R wave in V_3 in Figure 7.1). This pattern proved to be somewhat misleading in this instance. Often, this type of ECG pattern is present in idiopathic VTs/PVCs that originate from the epicardial aspect of the septum or the "crux of the heart." V_2 behaves discrepant to the adjacent leads possibly because it is closest to the septum. Therefore, the "pattern break" has been described for epicardial VTs from the anterior part of the heart (summit) and the posterior part of

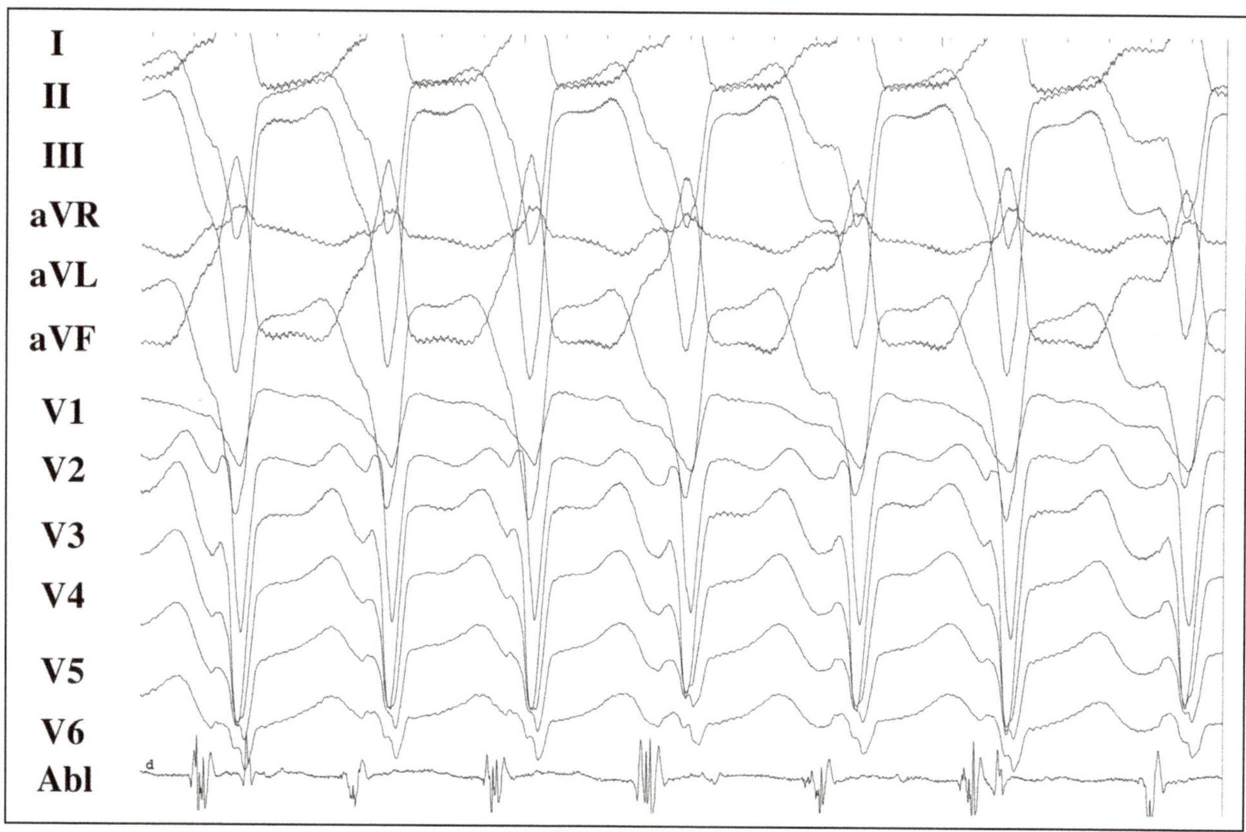

Figure 7.2 A 12-lead ECG of the induced VT with intracardiac recordings from the ablation catheter (Abl). The local activation time precedes the QRS complex by 50 ms.

the heart (crux). Mapping within the middle cardiac vein in this patient showed an activation time of −20 ms without matching pace map. Mapping of the tricuspid annulus showed an earlier activation time of −50 to −60 ms (**Figure 7.2**), as well as matching pace maps (**Figure 7.3**). The Q in the inferior leads indicates an inferior wall origin. All inferior leads are negative and show Q waves supporting that the arrhythmia originates from the inferior wall of the heart rather than the septum (**Figure 7.4**). However, lead III is more negative than II and aVF indicating that the activation originates from closer to the septum than the lateral RV free wall. Other available literature for tricuspid annular arrhythmias is not that helpful for localization of this particular VT.[2]

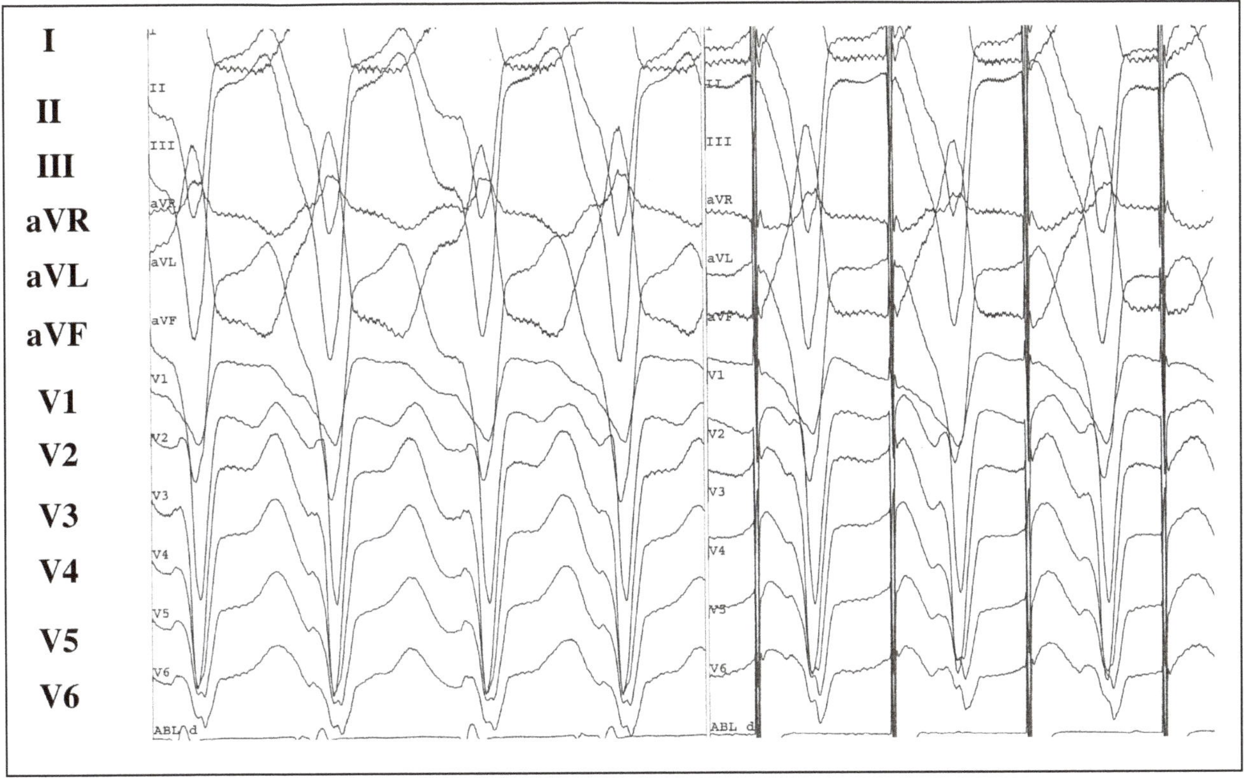

Figure 7.3   Pacing at this site shows a pace map with a similar QRS morphology and a stimulus-QRS complex of 60 ms.

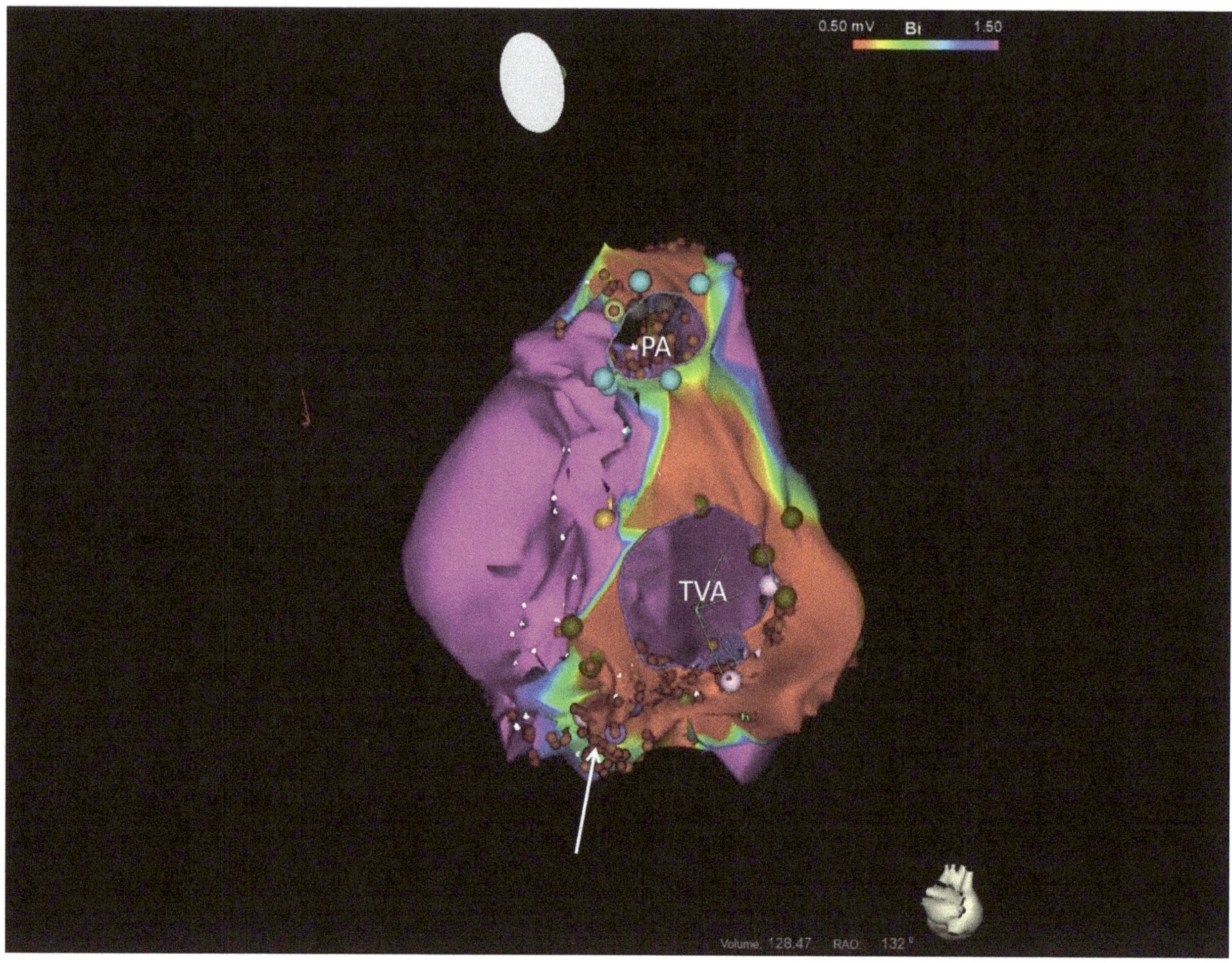

Figure 7.4 A bipolar voltage map of the posterior right ventricular endocardium. Indicated are the tricuspid valve annulus (TVA) and the pulmonary annulus (PA). Pacing and ablation (Figure 7.2 and Figure 7.3) was performed at the basal inferior tricuspid annulus (**arrow**) corresponding to areas of low voltage.

REFERENCES

1. Haqqani HM, Morton JB, Kalman JM. Using the 12-lead ECG to localize the origin of atrial and ventricular tachycardias: Part 2—ventricular tachycardia. *J Cardiovasc Electrophysiol.* 2009;20(7):825–832. PubMed PMID: 19302478.
2. Tada H, Tadokoro K, Ito S, et al. Idiopathic ventricular arrhythmias originating from the tricuspid annulus: Prevalence, electrocardiographic characteristics, and results of radiofrequency catheter ablation. *Heart Rhythm.* 2007;4(1):7–16. PubMed PMID: 17198982.

CLINICAL HISTORY

A 58-year-old woman with no history of prior medical illness, a structurally normal heart, and pectus excavatum presented for ablation of frequent, symptomatic PVCs and nonsustained VT. A year earlier, she had failed ablations with recurrent palpitations two days postablation. Imaging showed no evidence of structural heart disease.

Question

Where does the arrhythmia shown in **Figure 8.1** originate? Where would you map if there is difficulty in identifying the origin of this arrhythmia given that she had prior failed ablations?

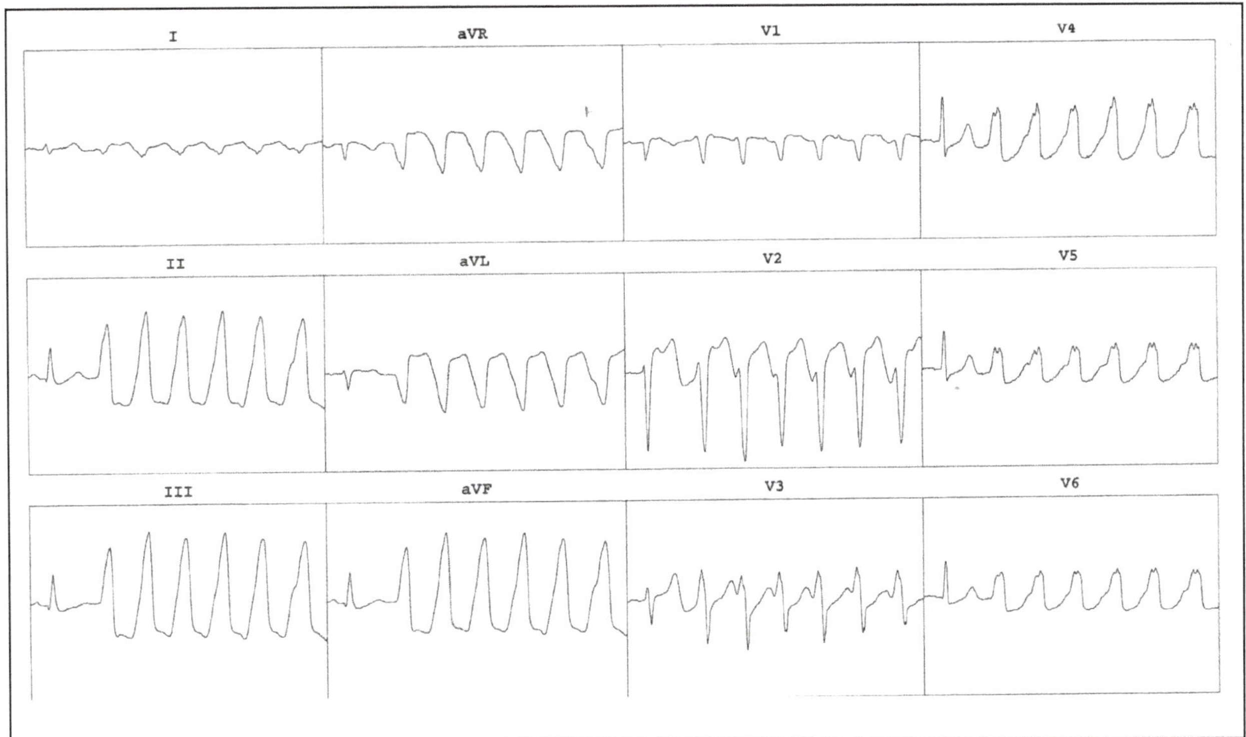

Figure 8.1 A 12-lead ECG of the patient's PVCs and VT.

Answer

The origin is the anteroseptal RVOT. The key findings here are: negative QRS in lead I indicating an anteroseptal origin because the RVOT is oriented towards the left, as opposed to the posterolateral RVOT that is oriented more towards the right, in which case lead I would be expected to be positive. The fact that the patient had a failed ablation procedure from within the RVOT does not rule out a RVOT origin.[1] In fact, the most frequent reason for a failed ablation procedure in a RVOT-like arrhythmia with a left bundle branch block inferior axis (LBBBIA) morphology is an origin in the RVOT that was missed during the prior procedure. The second most frequent and subsequent reasons for failed ablations are intramural origins, pulmonary artery origins, origin from the aortic cusps, and epicardial origins, being the least frequent origins identified. If the SOO of a ventricular arrhythmia with a LBBBIA morphology cannot easily be identified, these anatomic areas should be mapped carefully. **Figure 8.2** illustrates these different mapping areas, which were also mapped in this case.

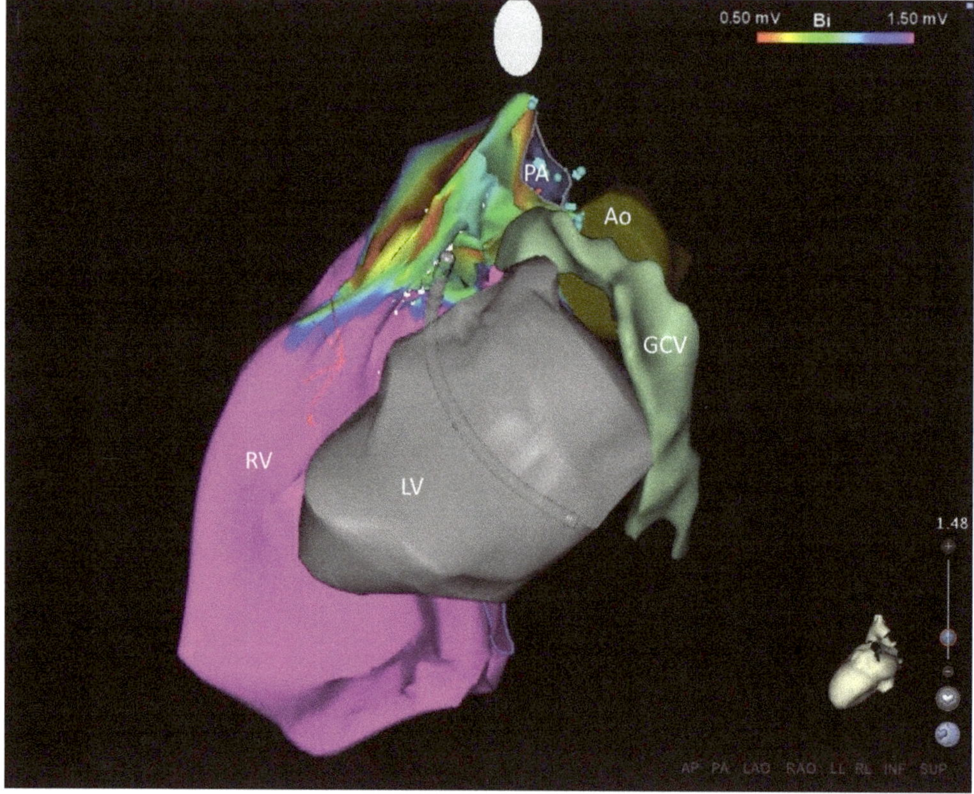

Figure 8.2   Voltage map of the septal aspect of the RVOT; there is low voltage in the RVOT close to the pulmonic valve. The low voltage is likely a result of the prior ablation lesions. Brown tags indicate ablation lesions and the catheter is shown at the site of successful ablation. The contours of the left ventricle (LV) and right ventricle (RV) are 3D reconstructions of the 2D echo contours, as is the aortic cusp (AC). The great cardiac vein (GCS) is part of the electroanatomic map reconstructed when the coronary venous system was mapped.

REFERENCE

1. Yokokawa M, Good E, Crawford T, et al. Reasons for failed ablation for idiopathic right ventricular outflow tract-like ventricular arrhythmias. *Heart Rhythm.* 2013;10(8):1101-8. PubMed PMID: 23702237.

CLINICAL HISTORY

A 62-year-old man presented with normal coronary arteries based on cardiac catheterization. The patient had an aortic aneurysm with status post-valve sparing aortic root replacement (36-mm graft). He has a preserved left ventricular function and abnormal heart by cardiac MRI. He presented with symptomatic PVCs despite beta-blocker therapy. The PVC burden ranged between 4%–8%.

Question

Where is the SOO of the arrhythmia shown in **Figure 9.1**? Are there any necessary precautions for ablation in this area?

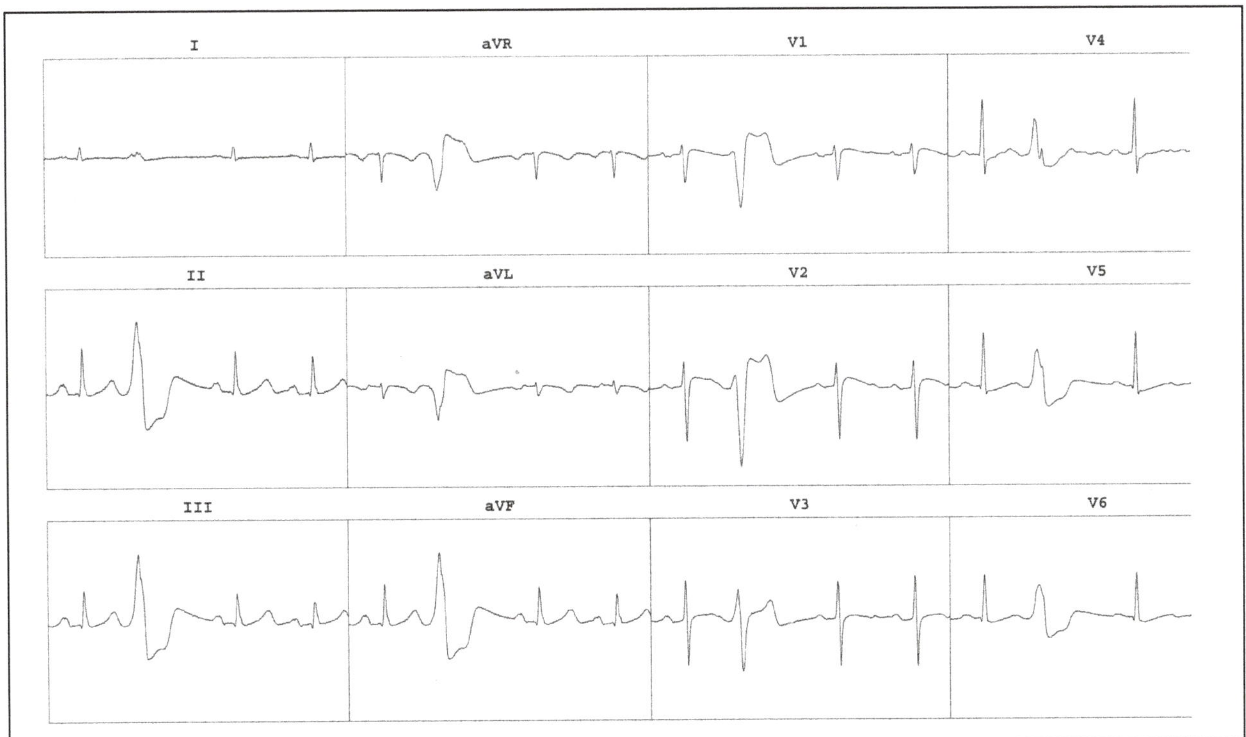

Figure 9.1   A 12-lead ECG showing the patient's arrhythmia.

Answer

The SOO is the PA. There are no ECG characteristics that clearly differentiate an origin from within the PA compared to other sites of the RVOT. Higher amplitudes in the inferior leads have been described; however, this is not helpful, because there is no absolute cut-off value from one patient to another. Pacing in the distal RVOT, below the pulmonic valve, most often reproduces the morphology of the arrhythmias regardless of whether the arrhythmias originates above or below the pulmonic valve. Therefore, it is not surprising that there are no good ECG criteria separating PA from other RVOT sites. A Q wave in lead I may indicate a possible supra-valvular origin: i.e. a more leftward and therefore higher position in the RVOT or the pulmonary artery, but this was not the case in this patient. Therefore, it is prudent to start the mapping procedure higher up in the PA and gradually withdraw the catheter into the RVOT

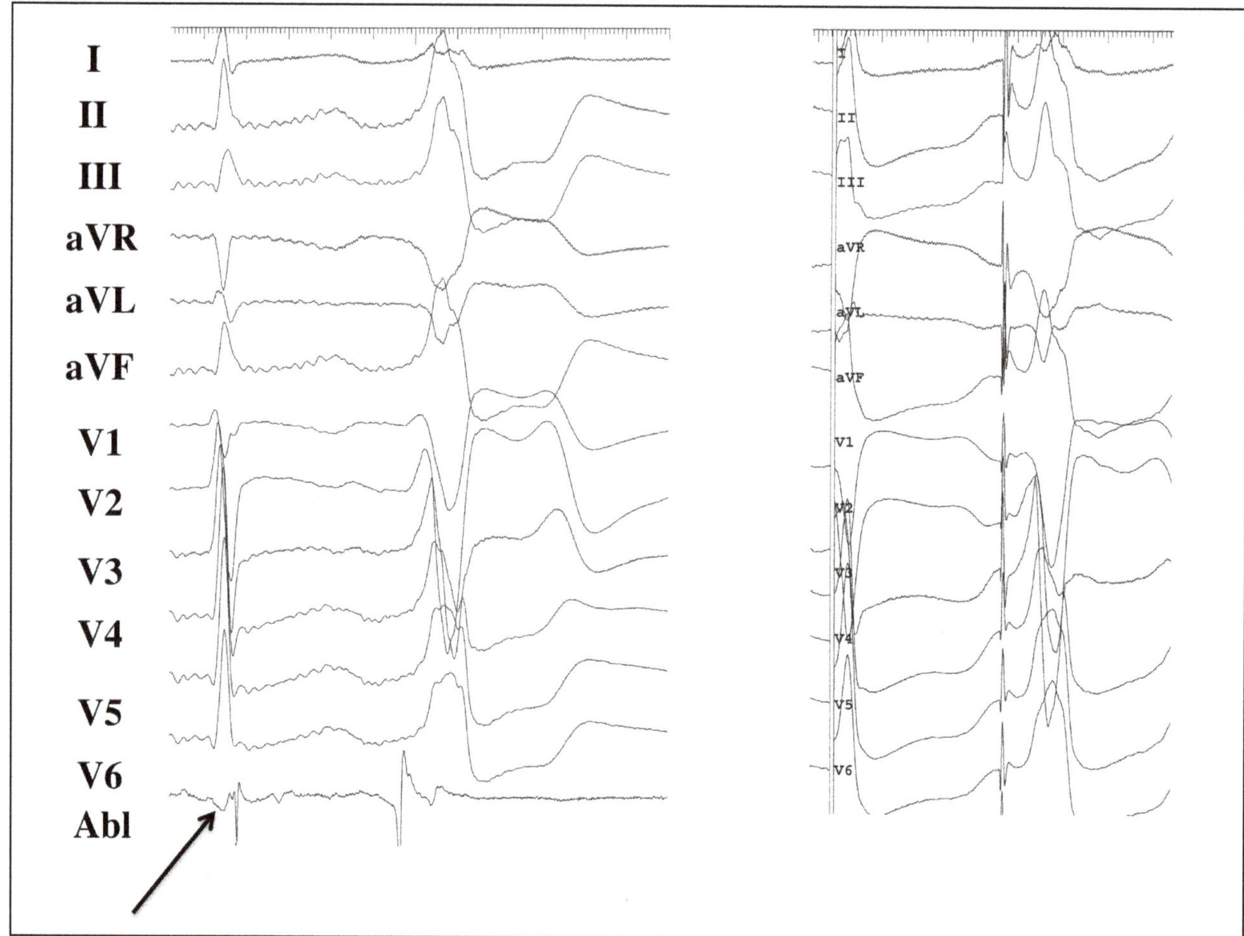

Figure 9.2 A 12-lead ECG with intracardiac tracings at the site of origin. **Left panel:** The activation time precedes the QRS onset of the PVC by 32 ms. Note the sharp ventricular potential during sinus rhythm (**arrow**). This indicates activation of a muscle sleeve extending above the pulmonic valve analogous to pulmonary vein potentials in the pulmonary veins. **Right panel:** The pace map at this site is similar, but not identical, to the targeted PVC morphology at the site of origin.

in all ventricular arrhythmias with a LBBB morphology with inferior axis in order to capture a PA origin. Ablation at the site of earliest RVOT activation often is ineffective and a cause of recurrences. One has to be careful when ablation in the PA is performed, given the close proximity of the left main coronary artery and the left anterior descending artery in some aspects of the PA, and hence reduction of power during RF delivery is important. Mapping above the pulmonic valve identified the earliest activation with an activation time of −32 ms (**Figure 9.2**). A sharp potential occurring late during sinus rhythm indicated the presence of extensions of muscle sleeves beyond the pulmonic valve similar to pulmonary venous potentials in the pulmonary veins. **Figure 9.3** shows the catheter location in the pulmonic artery, visualized with intracardiac echocardiography.

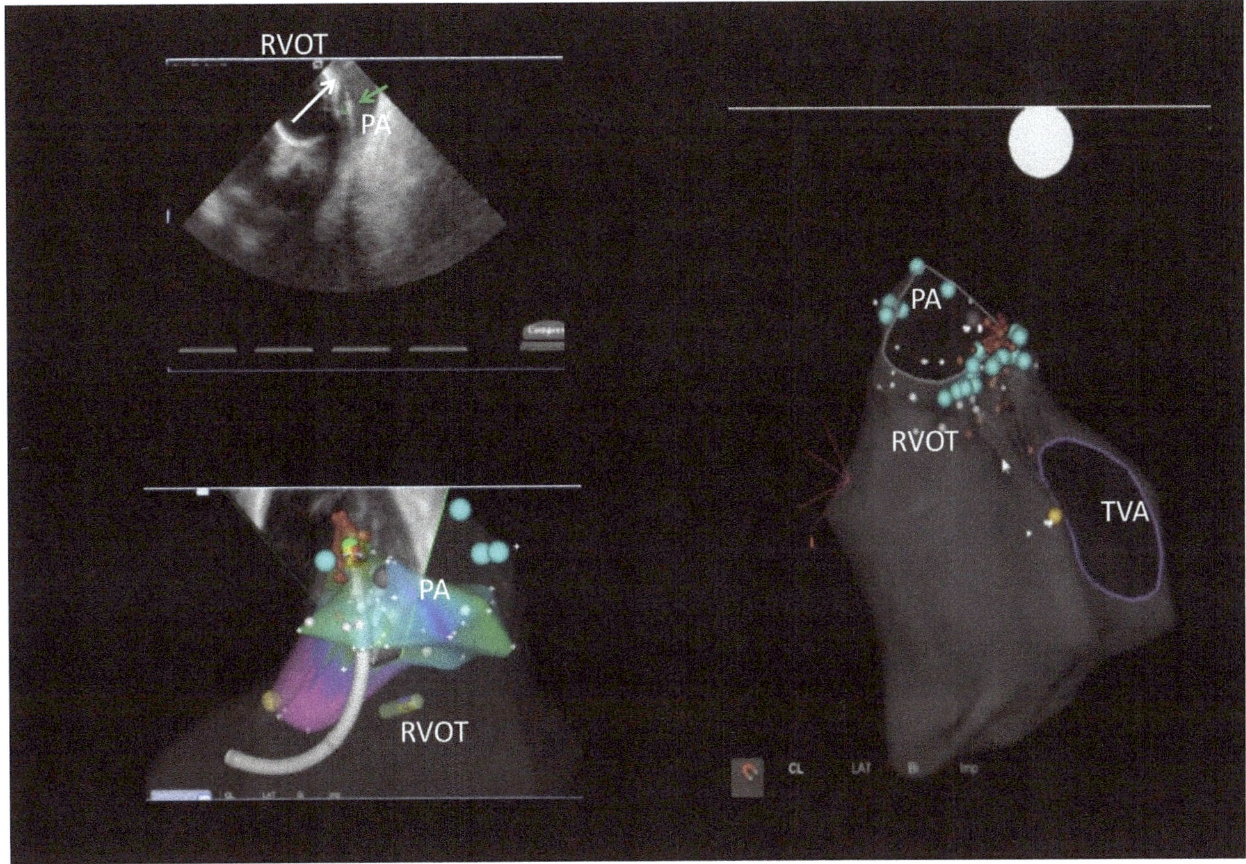

Figure 9.3 **Left top panel:** Intracardiac ultrasound displaying the RVOT, the level of the pulmonic valve (**white arrow**), and the location of the ablation catheter (**green icon** and **green arrow**) that is located above the pulmonic valve. **Left lower panel:** This figure shows an activation map with **blue dots** indicating the level of the pulmonic valve. The location of the ablation catheter is the same as in the insert in the top left panel. The 2D intracardiac echo plane displayed in the top left insert is shown in the 3D echo reconstruction. **Right panel:** Shown is the 3D reconstruction of the intracardiac echocardiographic contours from a posterior view showing the RVOT, the PA, and the tricuspid valve annulus (TVA). The **light blue tags** indicate the echocardiographic level of the pulmonic valve. The **red tags** indicate ablation lesions.

REFERENCE

1. Sekiguchi Y, Aonuma K, Takahashi A, et al. Electrocardiographic and electrophysiologic characteristics of ventricular tachycardia originating within the pulmonary artery. *J Am Coll Cardiol.* 2005;45(6):887–895. PubMed PMID: 15766825.

CLINICAL HISTORY

A 78-year-old woman had a pacemaker implantation for sinus node dysfunction. She had mitral valve repair for severe mitral valve prolapse and mitral valve regurgitation three years earlier. The patients presented with recurrent episodes of palpitations with presyncope. Her pacemaker interrogation shows high ventricular rate events with cycle lengths up to 260 ms lasting up to 15 beats. An ECG shows an ejection fraction of 45% with diffuse hypokinesis. There was no inducible ischemia during a nuclear stress test. A 12-lead Holter showed the following rhythm (**Figure 10.1**). **Figure 10.2** shows three segments of an intracardiac ECG obtained after placing the echo probe into the RVOT. The first image shows the LV septum and apex, slices 2 and 3 are obtained with more clockwise rotation of the echo probe.

Question

Where is the SOO of the arrhythmia shown in Figure 10.1?

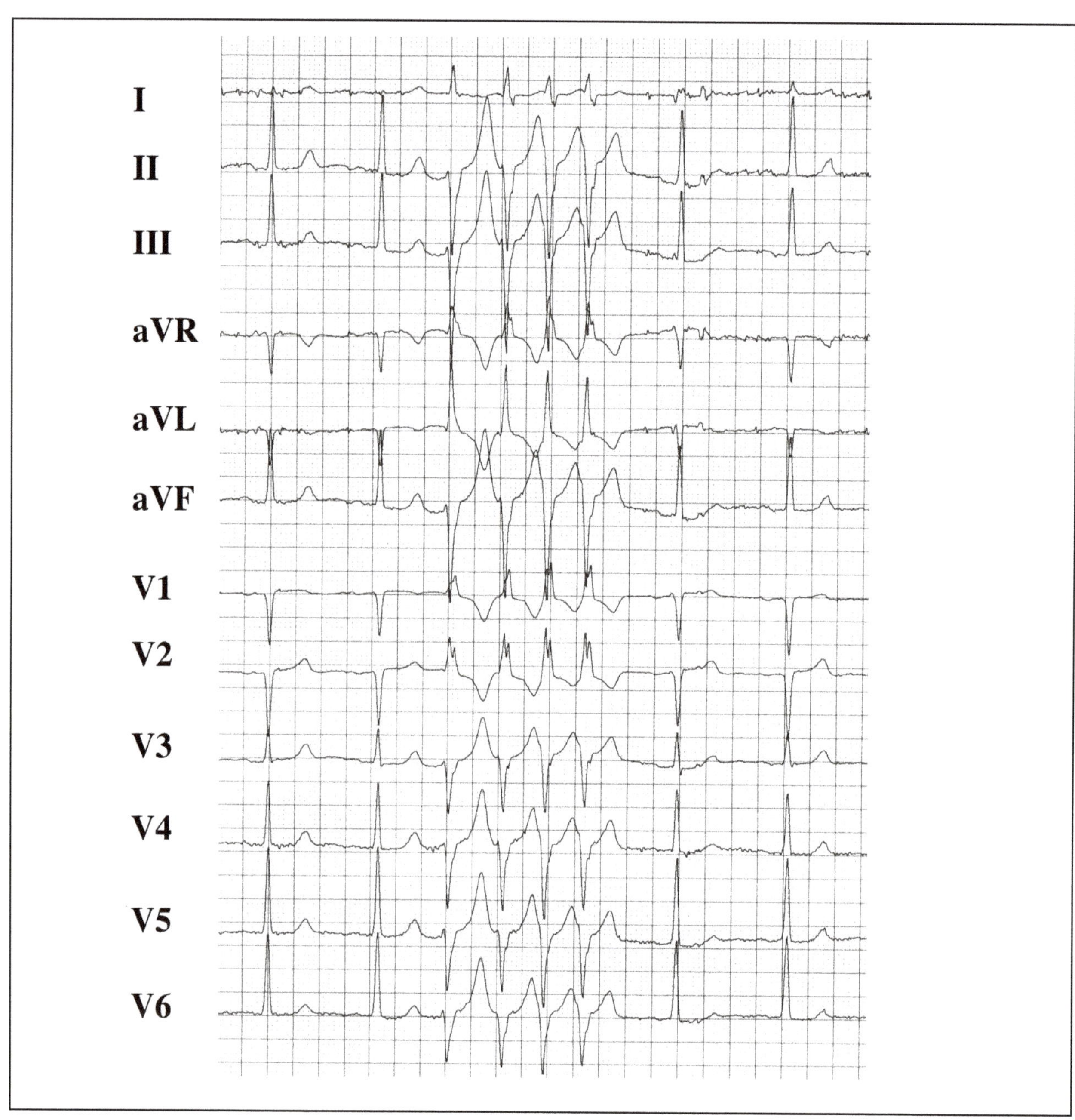

Figure 10.1 A 12-lead ECG from a 12-lead Holter monitor recording.

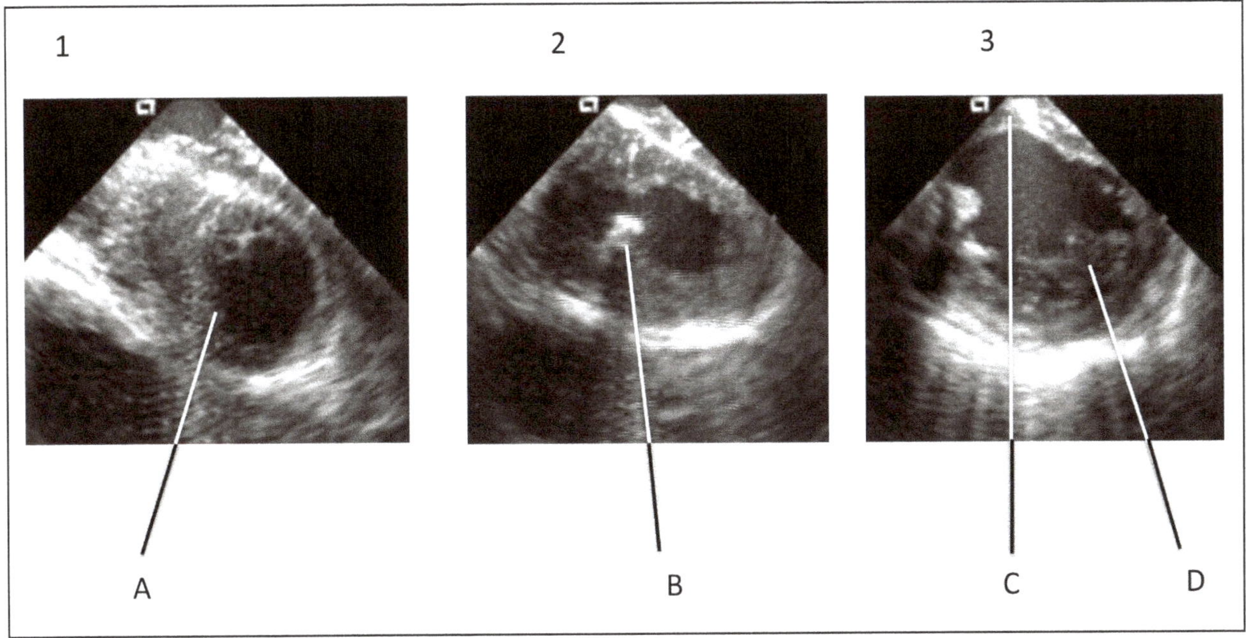

Figure 10.2   Three short-axis views from an intracardiac echo probe inserted into the RVOT. **Left panel:** Paraseptal short-axis view. **Middle panel:** This shows the body of the posteromedial papillary muscle that is calcified at the tip. **Right panel:** Basal left ventricle with the anterolateral papillary muscle.

Answer

The arrhythmia originated from the posterior fascicle (site A). Site A shows the posteroseptum of the LV. The ECG hints are the narrow QRS complex and the typical morphology of a fascicular arrhythmia originating from the posterior fascicle.[1,2] An ablation of the posterior fascicle eliminated her arrhythmias. Arrhythmias from the posteromedial papillary muscle (site B) have a broader QRS complex with a mean QRS width of 150 ms as compared to ventricular arrhythmias originating from the fascicles, which had a mean QRS width of 127 ms.[1] In this case, the QRS width here is 120 ms. Furthermore, fascicular arrhythmias originating from the posterior fascicles have discrete q waves in the lateral limb leads (I and aVL); these q waves are usually absent in papillary muscle arrhythmias. Site C is the basal left ventricle and would have a broader QRS with positive concordance in the left precordial leads. Site D is the anterolateral papillary muscle, and ventricular arrhythmias originating from there would display an inferior axis.

REFERENCES

1. Good E, Desjardins B, Jongnarangsin K, et al. Ventricular arrhythmias originating from a papillary muscle in patients without prior infarction: A comparison with fascicular arrhythmias. *Heart Rhythm.* 2008;5:1530–1537.
2. Al'Aref SJ, Ip JE, Markowitz SM, et al. Differentiation of papillary muscle from fascicular and mitral annular ventricular arrhythmias in patients with and without structural heart disease. *Circ Arrhythm Electrophysiol.* 2015;8:616–624.

CLINICAL HISTORY

A 40-year-old woman with a history of remote myocardial infarction (MI) and implantable cardio-verter-defibrillator (ICD) placement presented with recurrent ventricular tachycardia (VT). Her ejection fraction was 25% with an apical aneurysm. She had recurrent monomorphic VT and ICD therapies despite amiodarone and mexiletine therapy.

Question

The 12-lead ECG for one of the induced arrhythmias is shown in **Figure 11.1**. What is the origin of this rhythm?

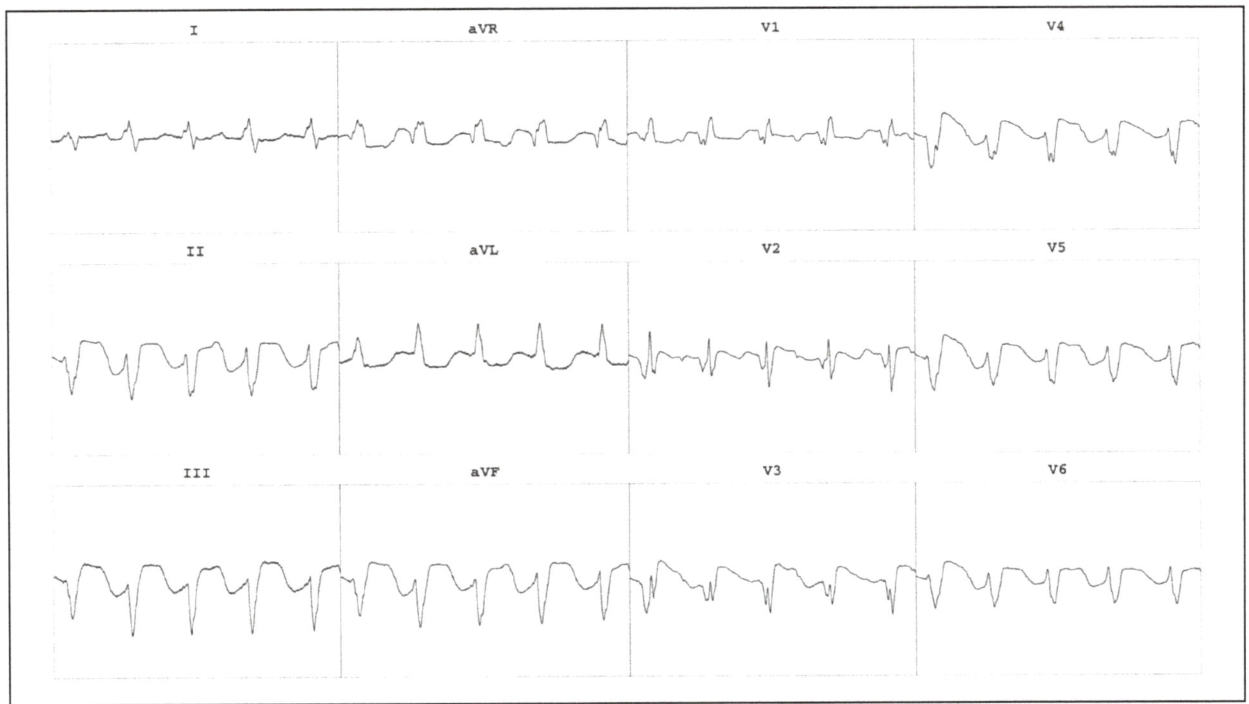

Figure 11.1   A 12-lead ECG of the patient's VT.

This is a fascicular VT originating from the posterior fascicle within scar tissue. The circuit involves both myocardial scar and the fascicular system. Therefore, the morphology is not the same as that of an idiopathic fascicular tachycardia: rsR' and narrow QRS and R/S transition in leads V_3/V_4 with discrete q waves in leads I and aVL. The Purkinje fibers are located in the septal scar and the QRS morphology is impacted by the scar location: q waves in leads V_1–V_2 indicating a septal origin; the absence of Q waves in the inferior leads indicate the absence of an inferior scar in this patient. Often

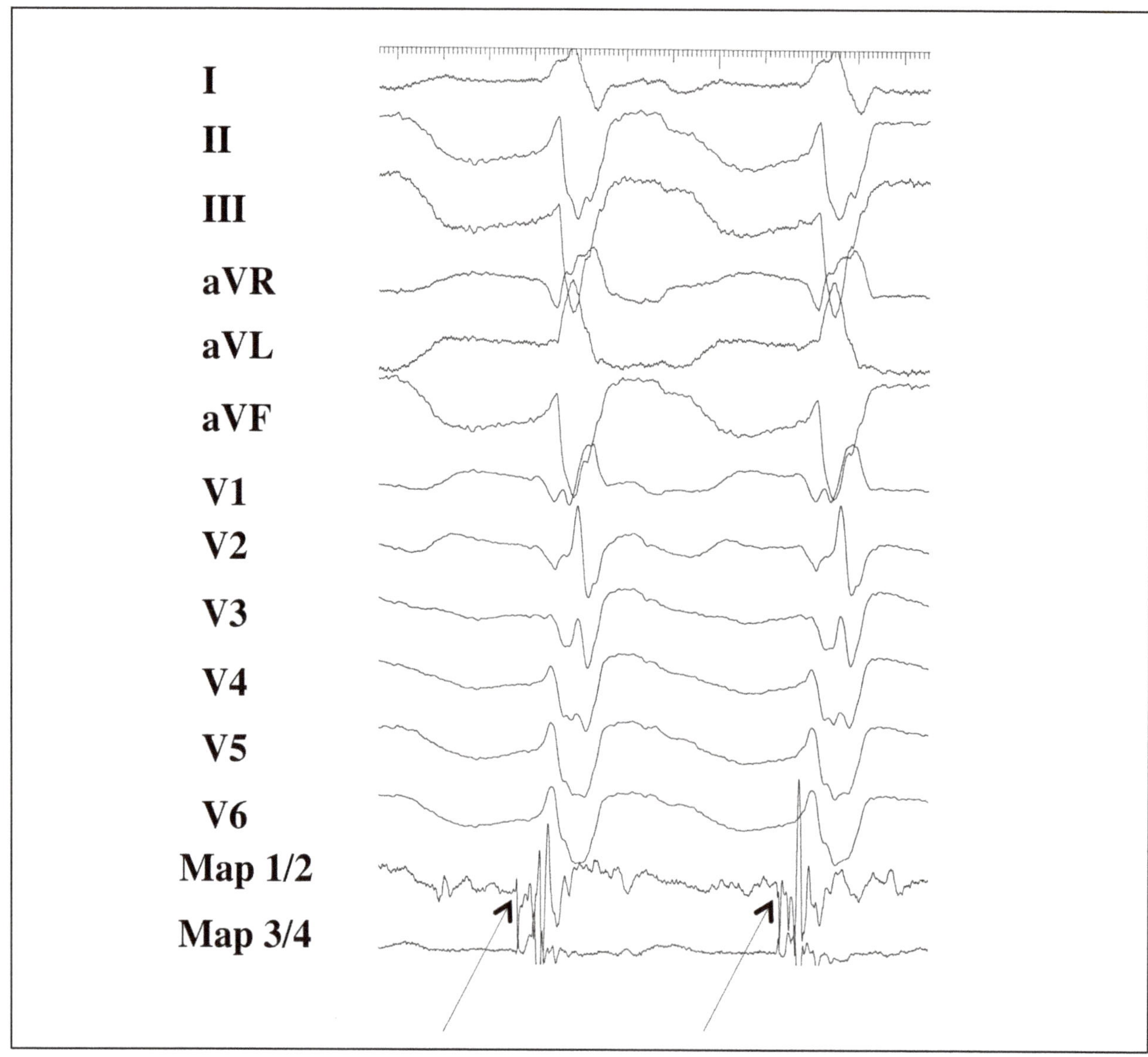

Figure 11.2 Intracardiac tracings of the site where Purkinje potentials were recorded during sinus rhythm and where VT was successfully ablated during sinus rhythm (**arrow**).

in patients with post–MI fascicular VT, there is an inferior wall scar. Hence, there are Q waves in the inferior leads, as in the example provided in the reference.[1] The QRS is relatively narrow, and this is still the main clue for a fascicular post–MI VT.[1] An intramural origin might also have a QRS that is narrower than endocardial postinfarction VTs. The leftward axis indicates that the posterior fascicle is involved. The ablation was performed at a site with Purkinje potentials during VT and during sinus rhythm (**Figure 11.2** and **Figure 11.3**), and there was a decent, but not perfect, pace map at the ablation site that eliminated VT.

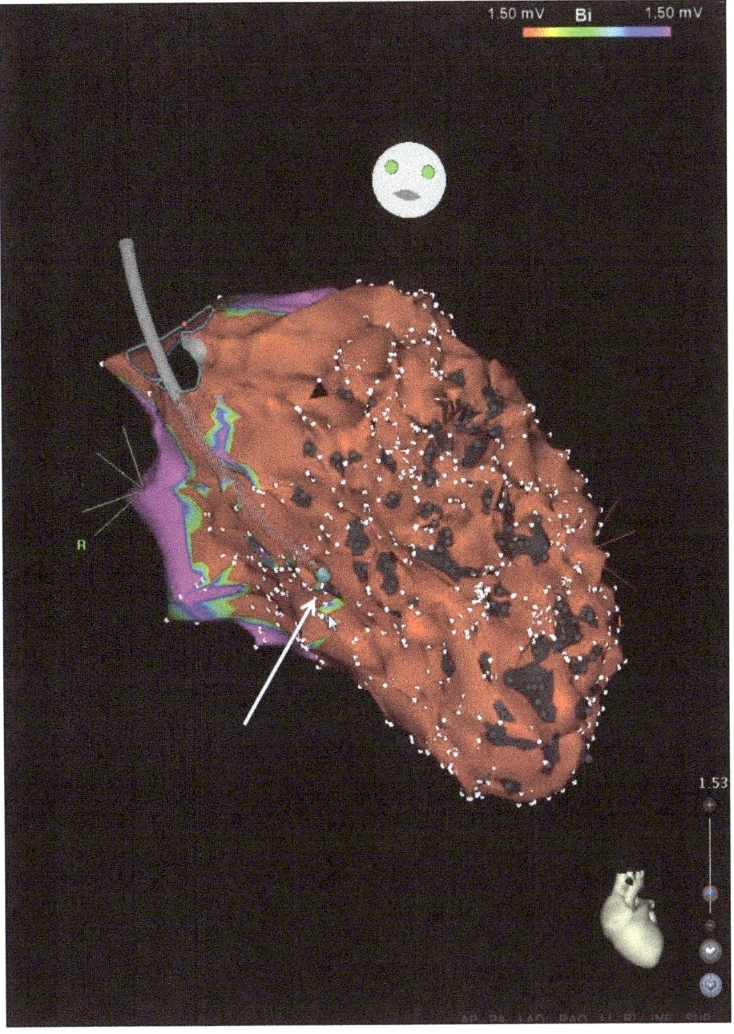

Figure 11.3 Lateral view of the voltage map of the left ventricle showing a large anteroseptal scar with the ablation catheter located at the site where the tracings from Figure 11.2 were obtained (**blue tag**). Ablation was performed at this site (**arrow**).

REFERENCE

1. Yoshida K, Yokokawa M, Desjardins B, et al. Septal involvement in patients with post-infarction ventricular tachycardia: Implications for mapping and radiofrequency ablation. *J Am Coll Cardiol.* 2011;58:2491–2500.

CLINICAL HISTORY

A 67-year-old woman presented with a history of recurrent VT and several failed ablation procedures. The patient was diagnosed with arrhythmogenic right ventricular cardiomyopathy and an endocardial/epicardial VT ablation was performed for her recurrent VTs after an ICD was implanted.

Question

Figure 12.1 shows one of the inducible VTs. Where is the origin?

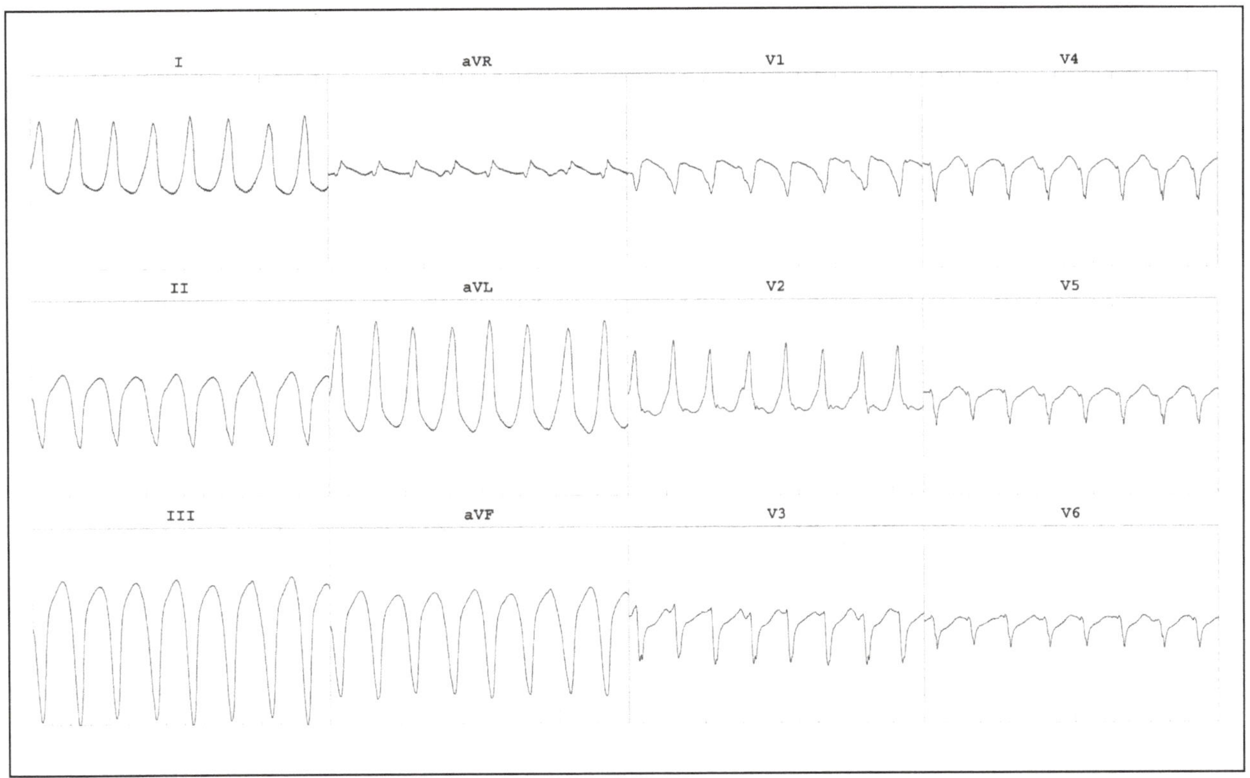

Figure 12.1   A 12-lead ECG showing the patient's VT.

Answer

The origin was the epicardial aspect of the basal inferoseptal myocardium. There is a rapid change from QS to Rs when going from V_1 to V_2 and back to an rS pattern in lead V_3. The term "pattern break" has been used for this observation.[1] The VT was mapped to the epicardial inferoseptal area where a matching pace map was identified (**Figure 12.2**), and RF ablation eliminated the VT (**Figure 12.3**).

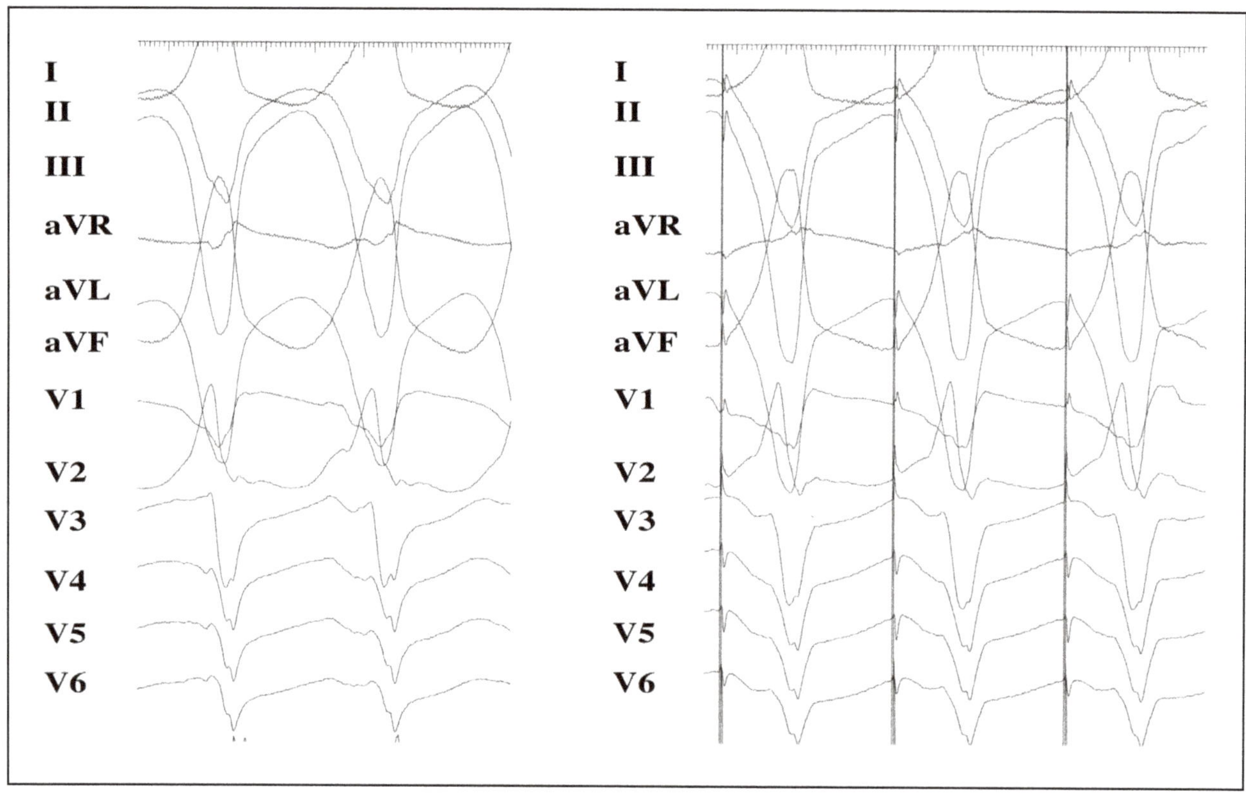

Figure 12.2   This figure shows a matching pace map in the inferior septal epicardium (**right panel**) with the induced VT (**left panel**).

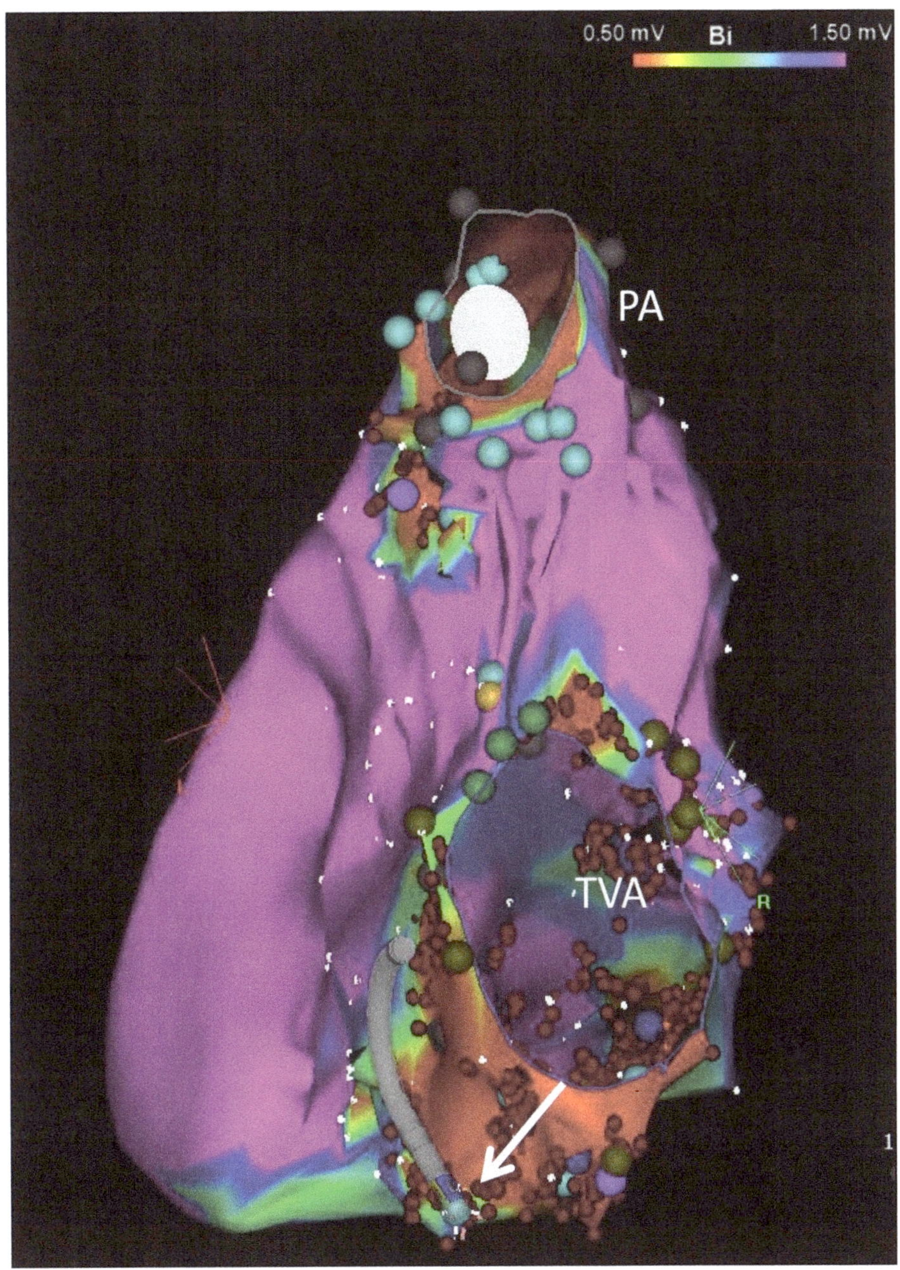

Figure 12.3 Electroanatomic voltage map of the posterior right ventricle. It features an inferobasal scar and the catheter location (**white arrow**) at the effective ablation site where the electrograms from Figure 12.2 were shown. The pulmonary artery and the tricuspid valve annulus (TVA) are indicated.

REFERENCE

1. Haqqani HM, Morton JB, Kalman JM. Using the 12-lead ECG to localize the origin of atrial and ventricular tachycardias: Part 2—ventricular tachycardia. *J Cardiovasc Electrophysiol.* 2009;20:825–832.

CLINICAL HISTORY

A 68-year-old man presented with a normal ejection fraction of 55% and mild LV dilatation (LV end diastolic dimension: 58 mm). He was found to have asymptomatic PVCs at time of colonoscopy. He underwent a cardiac MRI that showed no delayed enhancement. On two 24-hour Holter recordings, his PVC burden was 16.4% and 6.9%. The patient was referred for ablation.

Question

Figure 13.1 shows a couplet with two different PVC morphologies. Where do the two PVCs originate?

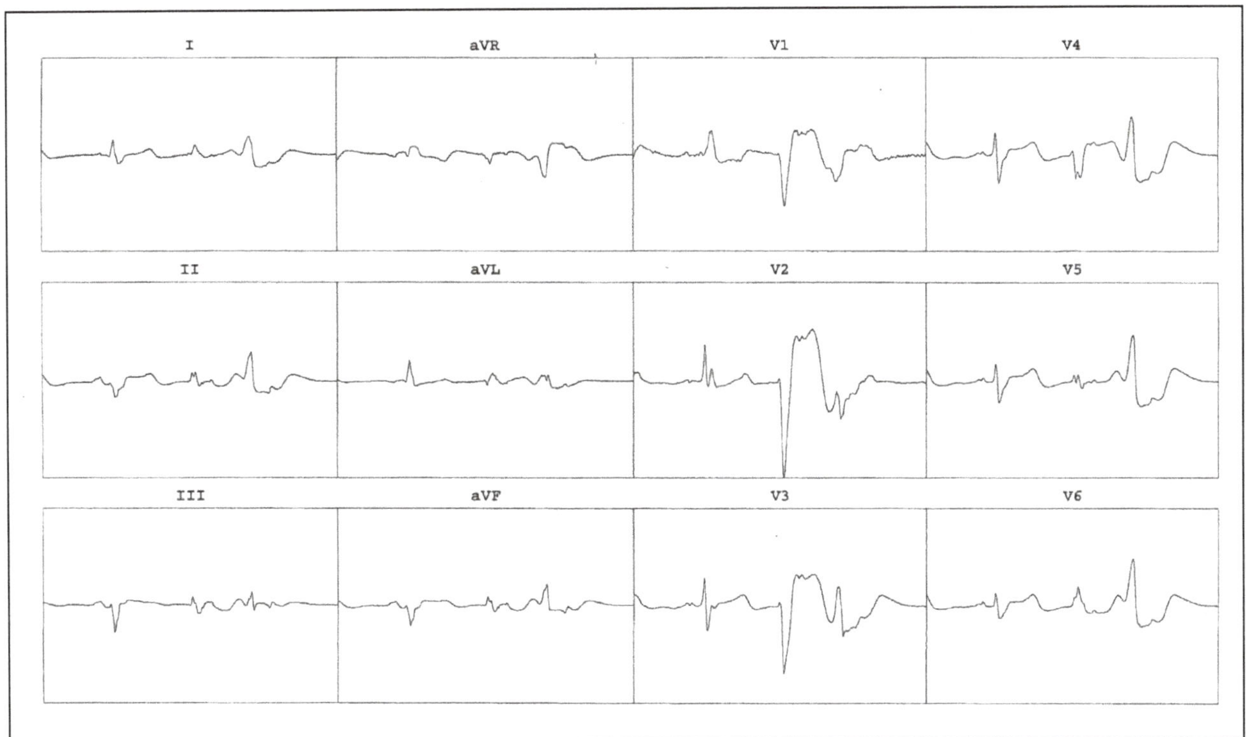

Figure 13.1 A 12-lead ECG of a PVC couplet.

The first PVC was mapped to the moderator band and the anterior papillary muscle insertion. This is where we had the best pace map. The patient had a complete right bundle branch block (RBBB) during sinus rhythm. At a site where we expected the right bundle branch to be located, about 2 cm distal to the His bundle location, in the mid-septum, we recorded on several occasions a sharp potential preceding the PVC but not during sinus rhythm (−35 ms, **Figure 13.2** and **Figure 13.3**). There was no matching pace map at this location, suggesting that there might have been myocardial capture at this site (also no change in QRS morphology with lower output). An ablation lesion eliminated the PVC. The Purkinje potentials most likely were a reflection of Purkinje fiber

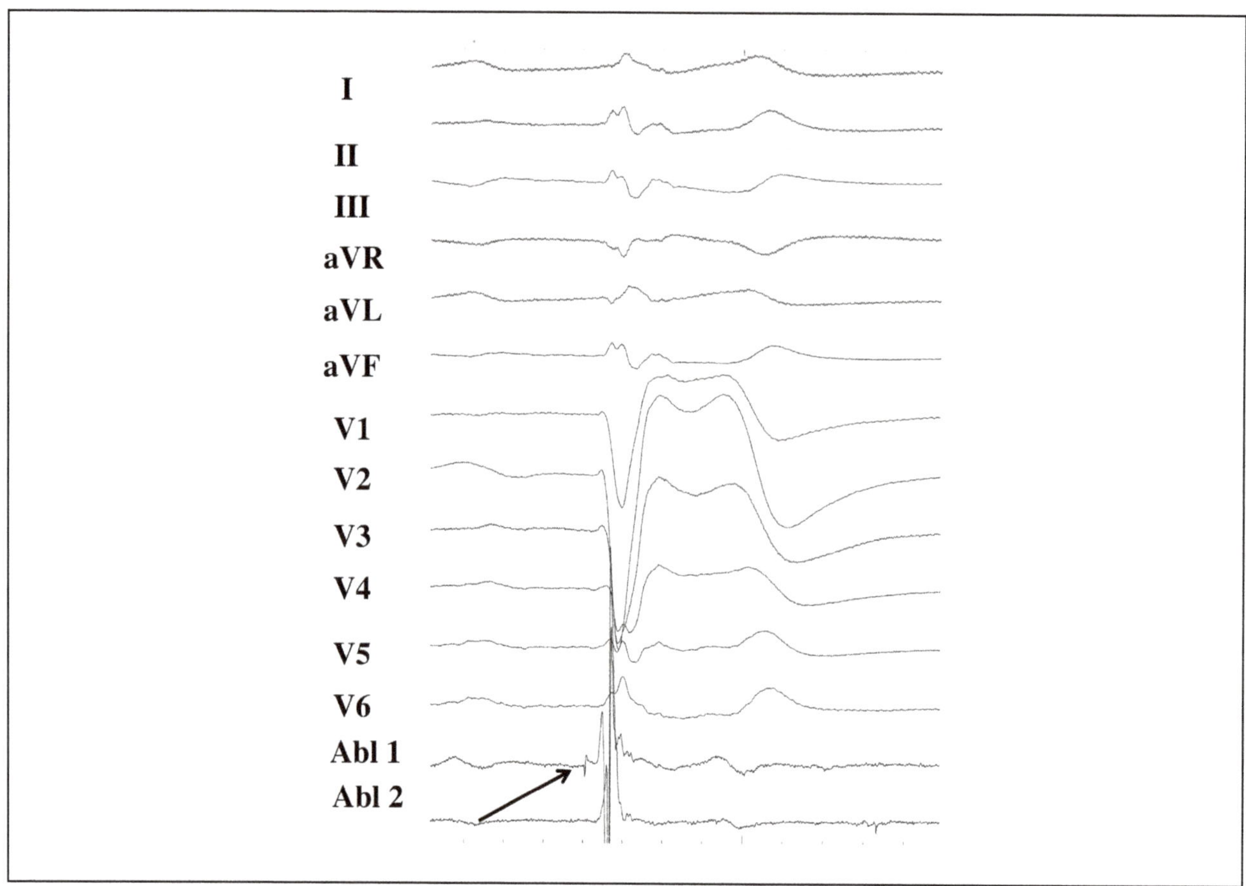

Figure 13.2 Tracings at the origin of PVC1. There is a Purkinje potential (**arrow**) indicating activity of the specialized conduction system during the PVC. Ablation at this site was ineffective due to catheter instability. At a slightly more distal site, ablation eliminated the PVC.

automaticity or triggered activity from the Purkinje fibers generating the PVC. Due to the complete RBBB, no Purkinje or fascicular potential was recorded during sinus rhythm. Further evidence in favor of a fascicular/Purkinje fiber origin was also the rapid initial activation of the QRS complex and the typical LBBB morphology. The late transition suggests a right ventricular (RV) origin. The second PVC was coupled to the first PVC and rarely occurred as a single PVC. Once the first PVC was ablated, the second PVC occurred sporadically without the first PVC as a single PVC. Unfortunately, the SOO was close to the His bundle and we were not able to ablate it. Hints for the parahisian location were the Q in V_1, a tall R wave in lead I, and a positive QRS in aVL.[1,2]

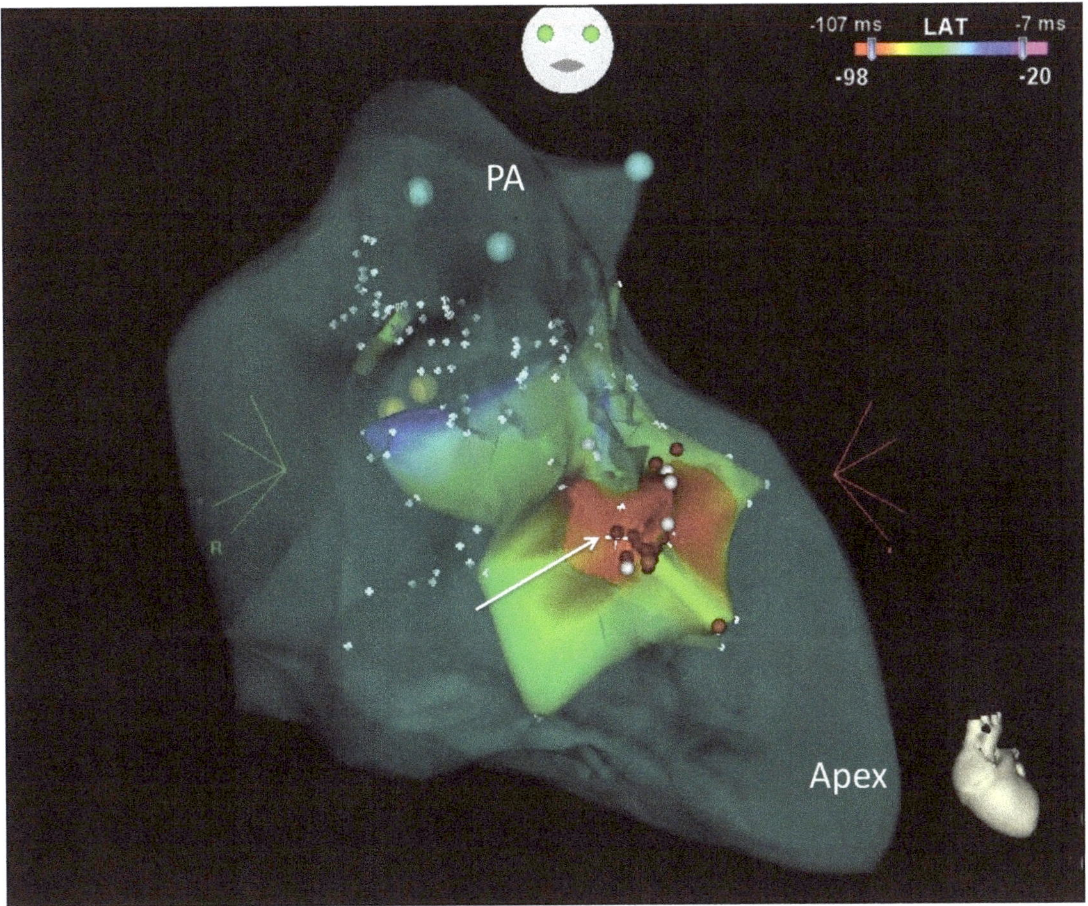

Figure 13.3 Electroanatomic activation map integrated into the 3D echocardiographic reconstruction of the right ventricle (**light green**) showing the right ventricle from an anterior aspect with the pulmonary artery and the right ventricular apex labeled. An **arrow** on the activation map indicates the site of origin, shown in Figure 13.2.

REFERENCES

1. Yamauchi Y, Aonuma K, Takahashi A, et al. Electrocardiographic characteristics of repetitive monomorphic right ventricular tachycardia originating near the his-bundle. *J Cardiovasc Electrophysiol.* 2005;16:1041–1048.
2. Tada H, Tadokoro K, Ito S, et al. Idiopathic ventricular arrhythmias originating from the tricuspid annulus: Prevalence, electrocardiographic characteristics, and results of radiofrequency catheter ablation. *Heart Rhythm.* 2007;4:7–16.

CASE
14

CLINICAL HISTORY

A 58-year-old woman with a history of nonischemic cardiomyopathy was diagnosed after she experienced sudden cardiac arrest in 2007. Her ejection fraction was 40% and she underwent placement of an ICD with cardiac resynchronization. She has a history of frequent PVCs, as well as, multiple sclerosis. Serial Holter monitoring showed a PVC burden between 18% to 35%. Mexiletine did not control her PVCs. A cardiac MRI did not show clear-cut delayed enhancement.

Question

Figure 14.1 shows the 12-lead ECG of the PVC. What is the SOO?

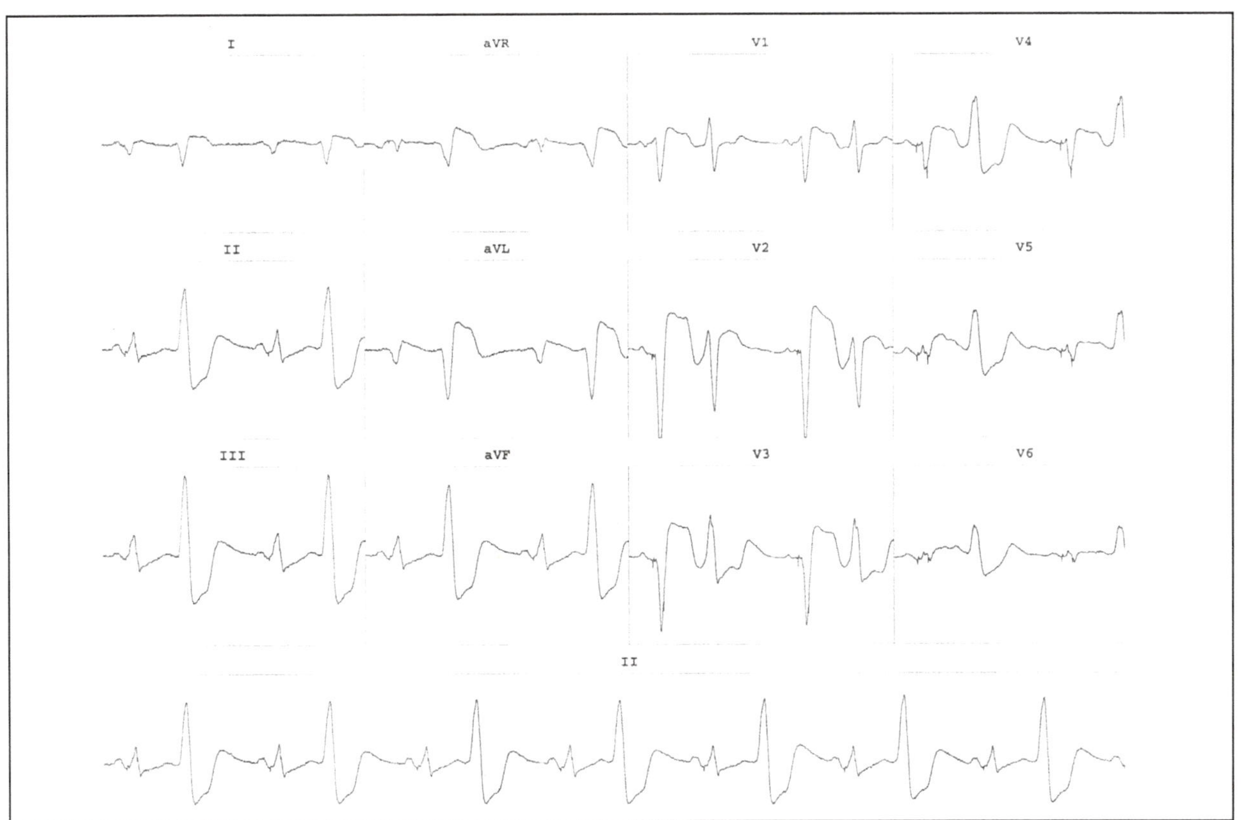

Figure 14.1 A 12-lead ECG with bigeminal pattern.

The origin was intramural in the high septum between the LVOT and RVOT. There are no published ECG criteria indicating an intramural origin. Ablation of intramural septal foci is difficult, but feasible.[1] Often, the diagnosis of an intramural origin is made after a long, ineffective mapping procedure. An intramural origin has been demonstrated to be present if PVCs can be temporarily suppressed by injection of cold saline (**Figure 14.2**) into the distal coronary sinus.[2] Other hints for an intramural origin are absence of a matching pace map at sites with early activation times and combination pace maps, making them better matches than single-site pace maps.[3] Based on the

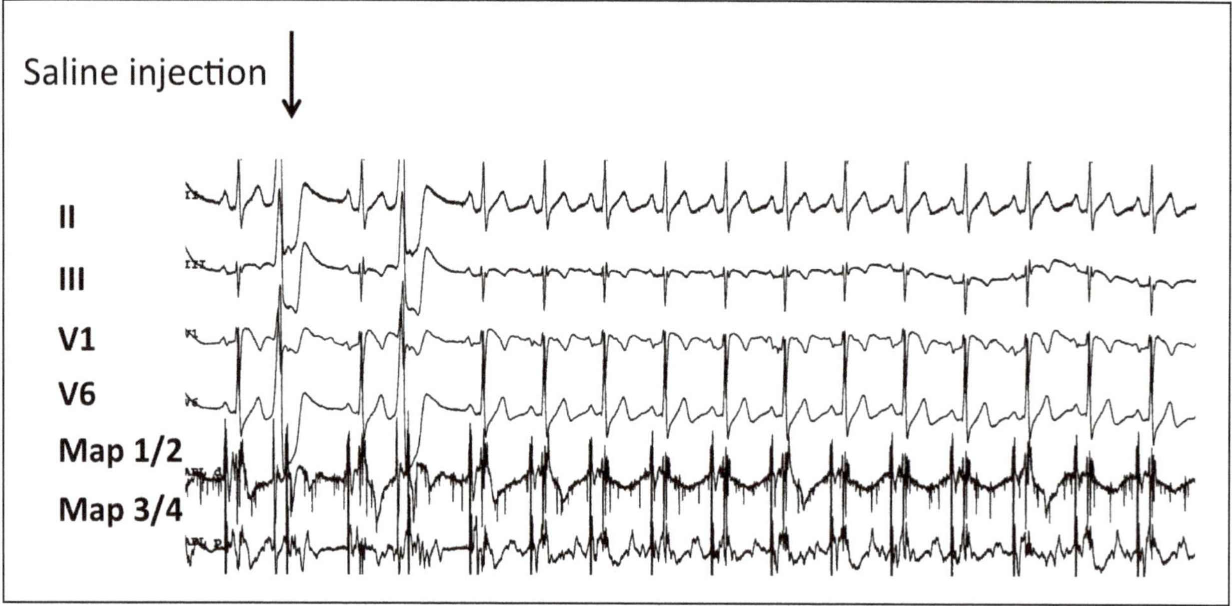

Figure 14.2   This figure shows the suppression of PVCs when cold saline was injected via the irrigated ablation catheter into the distal great cardiac vein.

morphology, an epicardial origin was also in the differential: broad R wave in V_1 and V_2 with a sizable S wave and a Q wave in lead I. However, the earliest timing in the anterior interventricular vein was −20 ms, similar to the earliest endocardial activation in the LVOT, the earliest site in the RVOT (**Figure 14.3**). Neither of these sites had a matching pace map, indicating that the origin was located deeper in the tissue. RF energy delivery from the left ventricular endocardium (after several lesions only) made the PVCs disappear permanently. RF energy was also applied from the RVOT and the coronary venous system (CVS); (**Figure 14.4**).

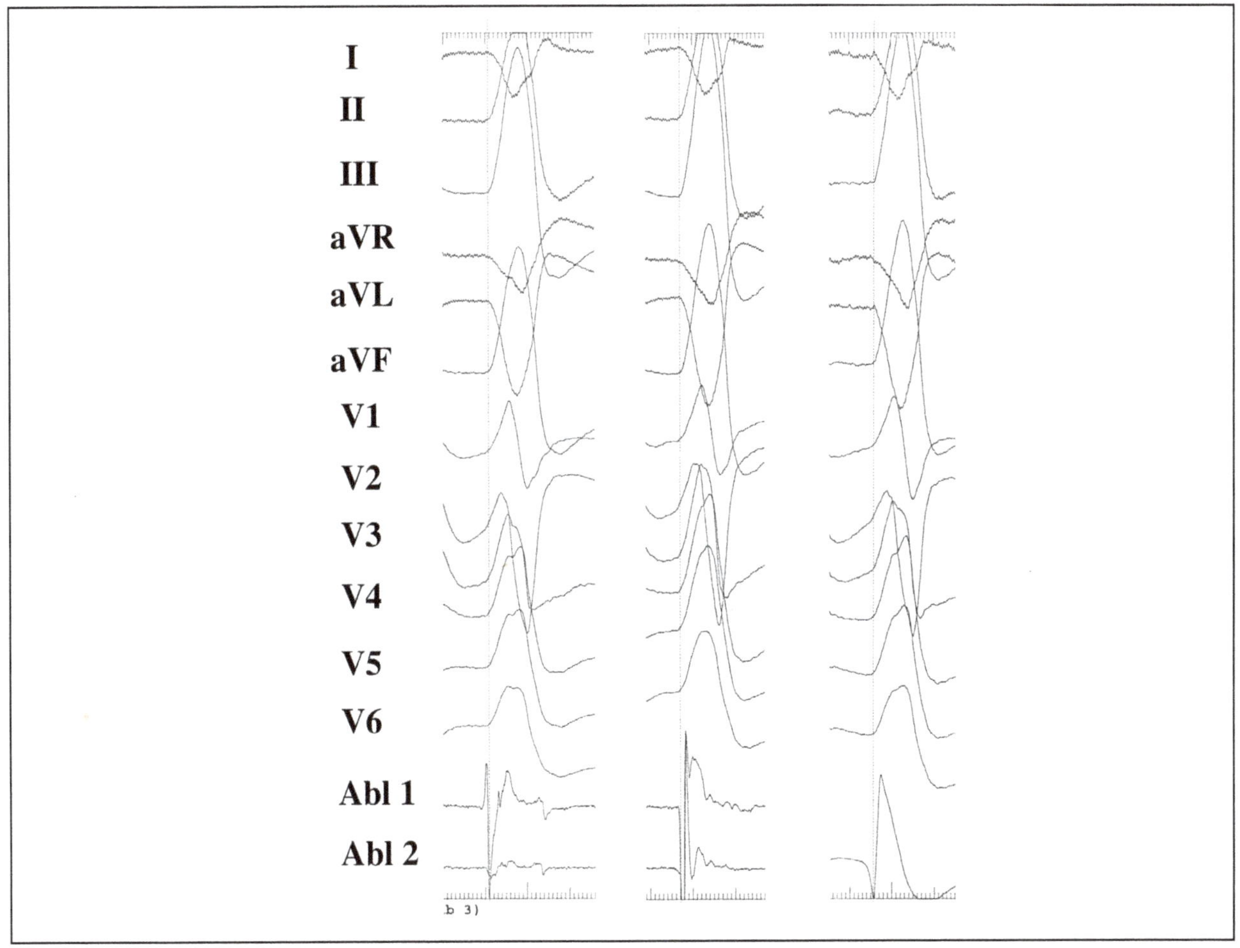

Figure 14.3   This figure shows the earliest activation times recorded in different anatomical areas, including the RVOT, the LVOT, and the CVS.

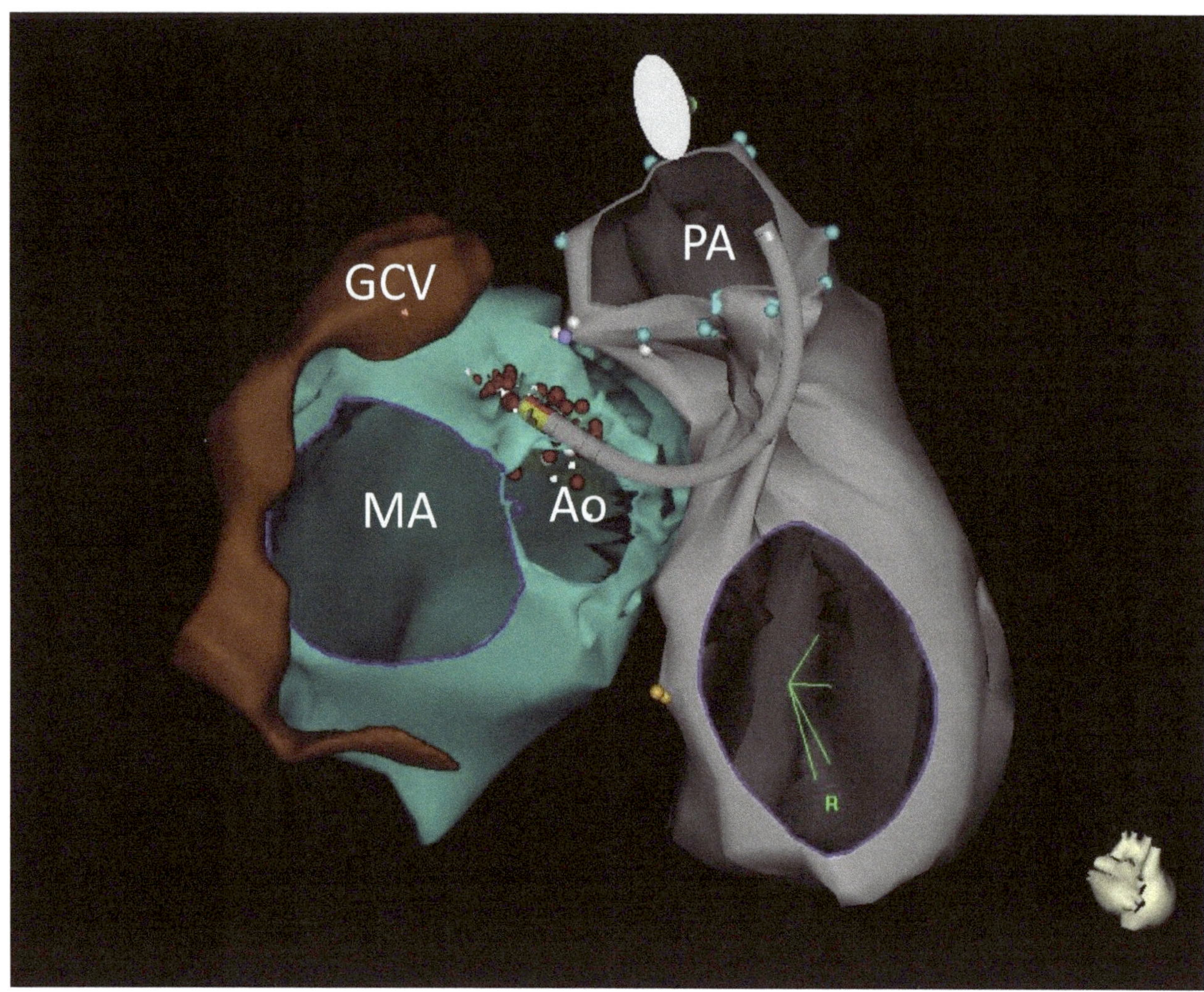

Figure 14.4   3D reconstruction of intracardiac echo images showing LV and RV from a posterior view. Indicated are the mitral valve annulus (MVA), the aortic cusp (Ao), the RVOT, and the great cardiac vein (GCV). Ablation lesions were delivered from the GCV, the LVOT, and the RVOT. The catheter is located at the MVA.

REFERENCES

1. Yokokawa M, Good E, Chugh A, et al. Intramural idiopathic ventricular arrhythmias originating in the intraventricular septum: Mapping and ablation. *Circ Arrhythm Electrophysiol.* 2012;5:258–263.
2. Yokokawa M, Morady F, Bogun F. Injection of cold saline for diagnosis of intramural ventricular arrhythmias. *Heart Rhythm.* 2016;13:78–82.
3. Yokokawa M, Yon Jung D, Hero AO, 3rd, Baser K, Morady F, Bogun F. Single- and dual-site pace mapping of idiopathic septal intramural ventricular arrhythmias. *Heart Rhythm.* 2016;13:72–77.

CLINICAL HISTORY

A 61-year-old man with hypertrophic cardiomyopathy and an ejection fraction of 35% presented with VT storm and multiple ICD shocks. During his electrophysiology procedure, 12 VTs were inducible. The VT shown in **Figure 15.1** is one of the 12 VTs. Preprocedural imaging with MRI showed extensive delayed enhancement involving the basal inferoseptal and inferior walls. The delayed enhancement was patchy and mid-myocardial. It also extended and involved the subepicardial aspect, particularly the inferoseptal and inferior walls, where it was transmural.

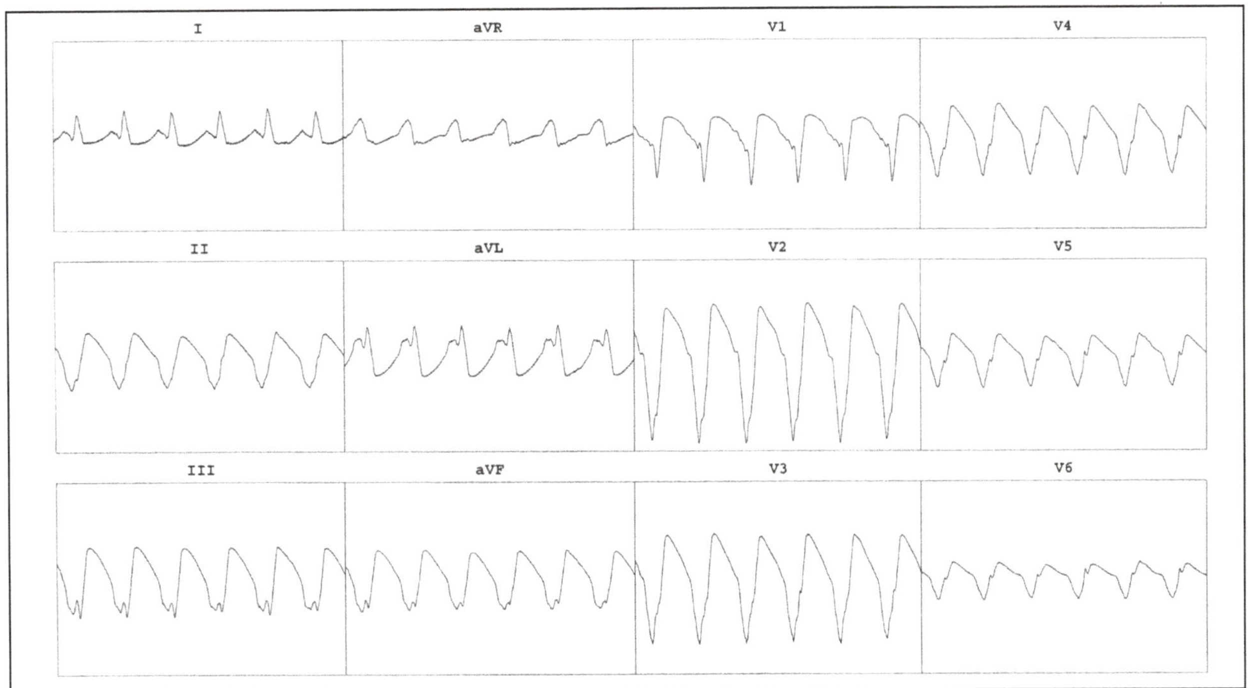

Figure 15.1   A 12-lead ECG of the patient's VT.

Question

Where does the VT shown in Figure 15.1 originate? **Figure 15.2** shows the VT of Figure 15.1 and a pace map generated by the ICD screw-in lead. What is the next best approach?

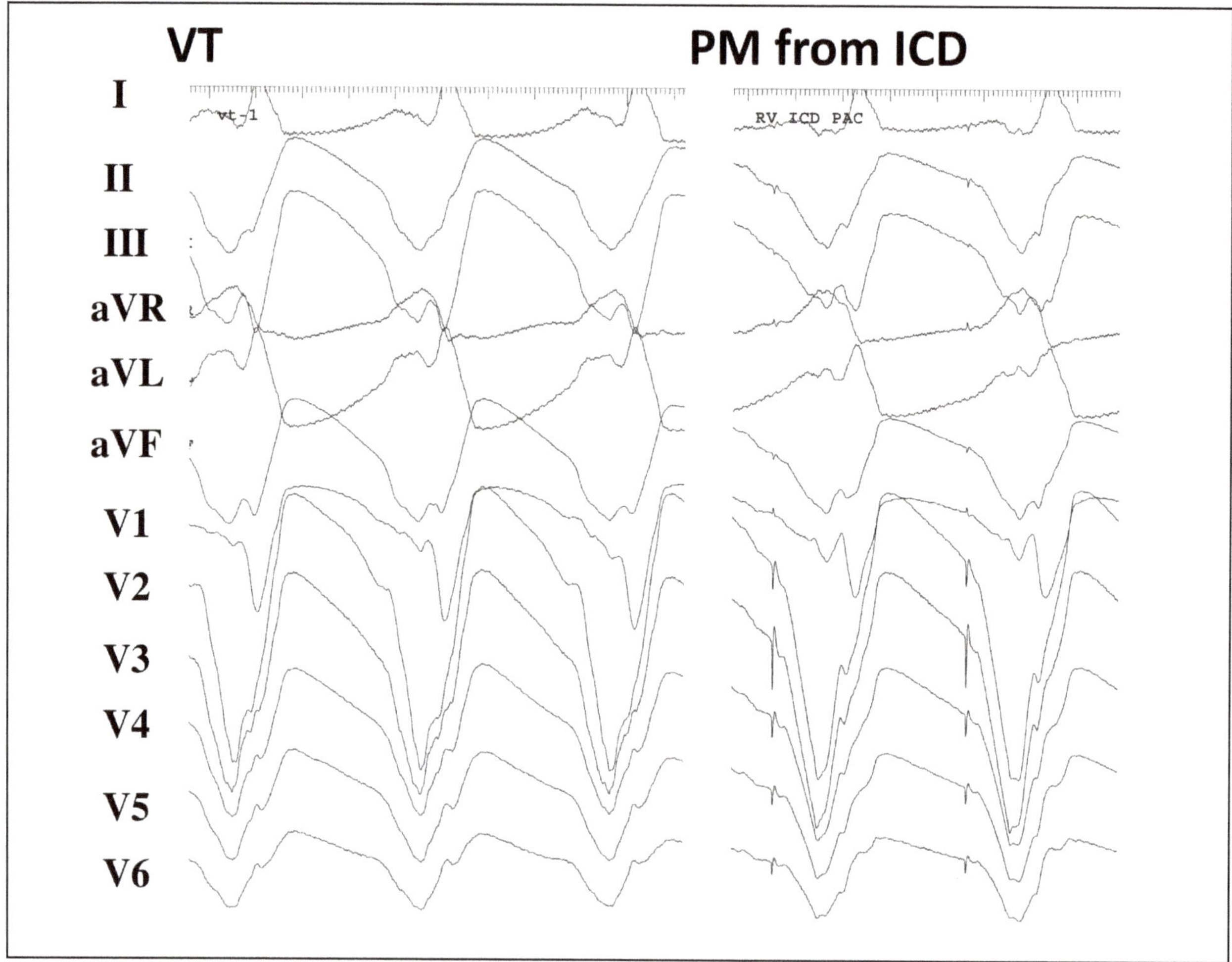

Figure 15.2 A 12-lead ECG of the induced VT (**left panel**) and pace map from the ICD lead that was located at the right ventricular (RV) apex. The morphology is similar.

Answer

An endocardial mapping/procedure failed to identify the origin of this VT. Pacing from the RV apex did not show a matching pace map for the VT shown in Figure 15.1. An epicardial procedure was subsequently performed.

The best pace map with short stimulus–QRS interval was from the location of the ICD lead located in the RV apex. This was seen only when pacing was performed from the ICD lead and not when pacing was performed from a lead adjacent to the ICD lead. The morphology is a LBBB with negative concordance and superior axis, possibly indicating an origin from the RV apex. RF energy was not delivered there given the lack of a matching pace map and the proximity of the ICD lead. In this patient, we mapped the epicardium and had a similar pace map (**Figure 15.3**) at a distance of about 2 cm away from the RV lead insertion at a site of transmural delayed enhancement (**Figure 15.4**). A hint for an epicardial origin in a patient without a transmural or epicardial scar is the absence of R waves in the inferior leads. The patient had an epicardial scar, suggesting that this would likely be the origin. The slower slope also indicates the possibility of an epicardial origin. One has to keep in mind that the origin of the paced QRS complex from the ICD lead is generated from deeper in the tissue, i.e., an intramural location, due to the intramural location of the screw. The scar in this patient extended from the intramural septum to the apical inferior epicardial wall (Figure 15.4, white arrow). Therefore, the most likely the origin is intramural, at a location between the best epicardial pace map and the location of the screw of the ICD lead. It is important to note that the stimulus-QRS interval from the epicardial pacing site is longer than the stimulus-QRS interval from the ICD lead, indicating that the exit site is somewhat remote from the epicardium. There are no described ECG criteria for intramural origins, but likely the slope is somewhere in between the slope of the endocardium and the epicardium.

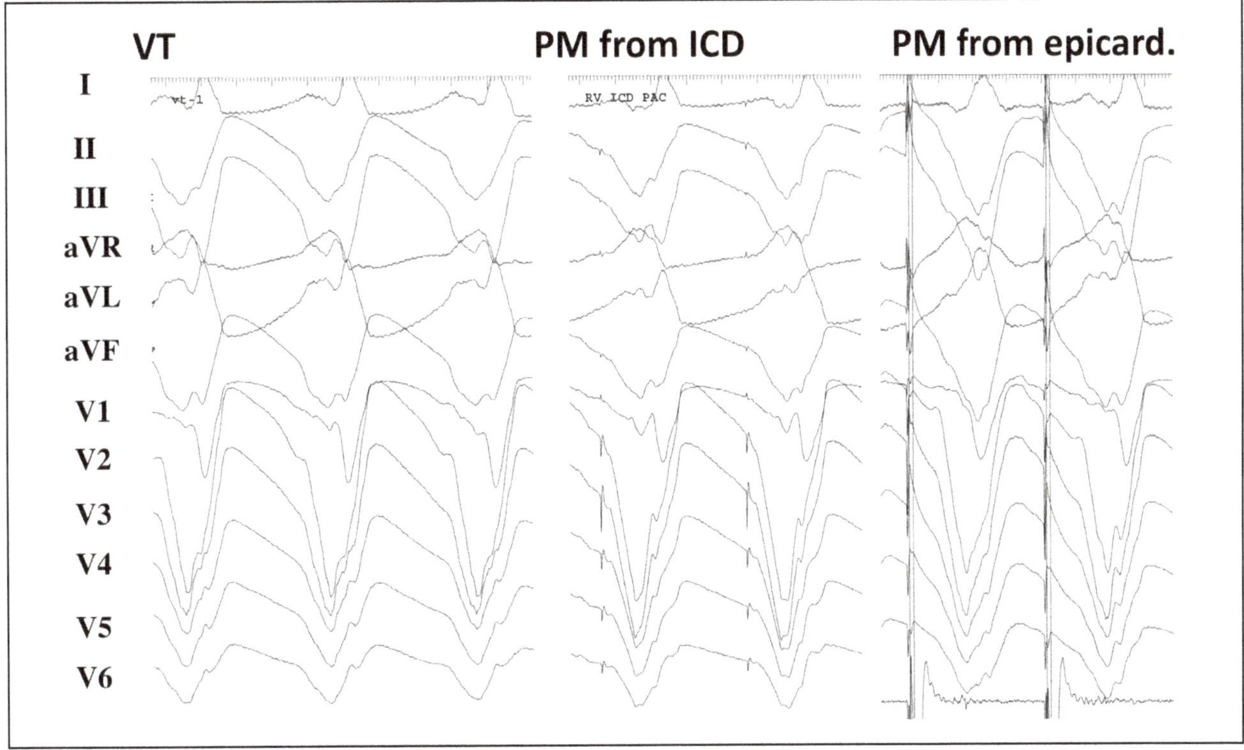

Figure 15.3 Tracings from Figure 15.2 and pace map from an epicardial site 2 cm away from the RV apex. There is a matching pace map (10/12 leads) with the clinical VT. There was low voltage at this site. Note that the stimulus-QRS interval is longer than the stimulus-QRS interval from the ICD lead.

One more thing to remember is that in patients with structural heart disease, ECG features are less specific for differentiating epicardial vs. endocardial origins/exit sites compared to patients without structural heart disease. Using only ECG features as a determinant for obtaining epicardial access would result in unnecessary epicardial procedures.[1–3] Other factors, such as imaging data, need to be considered, and moreover, intramural VT morphologies have not been factored into available algorithms.

VTs can also be generated as a result of ICD lead implantation, and the hallmark of this mechanism is a QRS morphology during antitachycardiac pacing that is identical to the QRS morphology of the VT. Often these arrhythmias are incessant and the treatment is repositioning of the ICD lead rather than ablation.

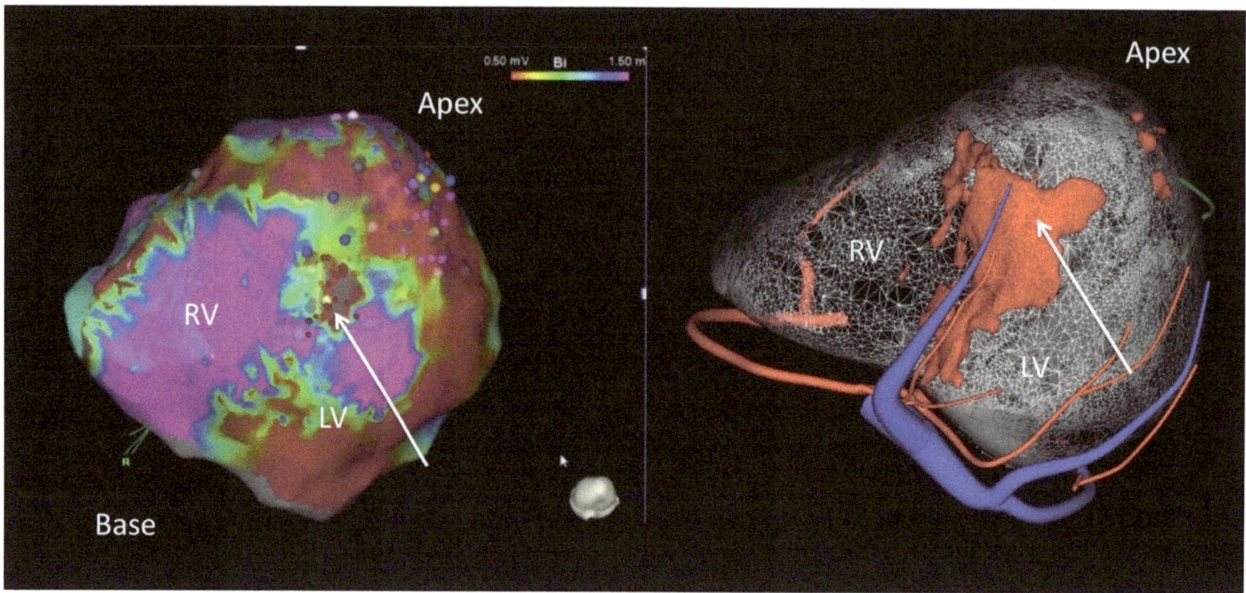

Figure 15.4　**Left panel:** Electroanatomic map of the basal apical RV. The site with a matching pace map where RF energy was delivered is indicated with a **white arrow**. **Right panel:** CT- and MRI-based reconstruction of the cardiac anatomy with MRI-defined scar (**red**) using the MUSIC software that was developed at the University of Bordeaux. The ablation site is indicated by a **white arrow**. Apex, the base of the heart, as well as RV and LV are indicated.

REFERENCES

1. Yokokawa M, Jung DY, Joseph KK, Hero AO, 3rd, Morady F, Bogun F. Computerized analysis of the 12-lead electrocardiogram to identify epicardial ventricular tachycardia exit sites. *Heart Rhythm.* 2014;11:1966–1973.
2. Berruezo A, Mont L, Nava S, Chueca E, Bartholomay E, Brugada J. Electrocardiographic recognition of the epicardial origin of ventricular tachycardias. *Circulation.* 2004;109:1842–1847.
3. Fernandez-Armenta J, Berruezo A. How to recognize epicardial origin of ventricular tachycardias? *Curr Cardiol Rev.* 2014;10:246–256.

CLINICAL HISTORY

A 43-year-old man presented with intractable palpitations and frequent PVCs. His PVC burden was 25% and his ejection fraction was 45%. There was no delayed enhancement in his cardiac MRI.

Question

Where is the origin of the PVCs in **Figure 16.1**?

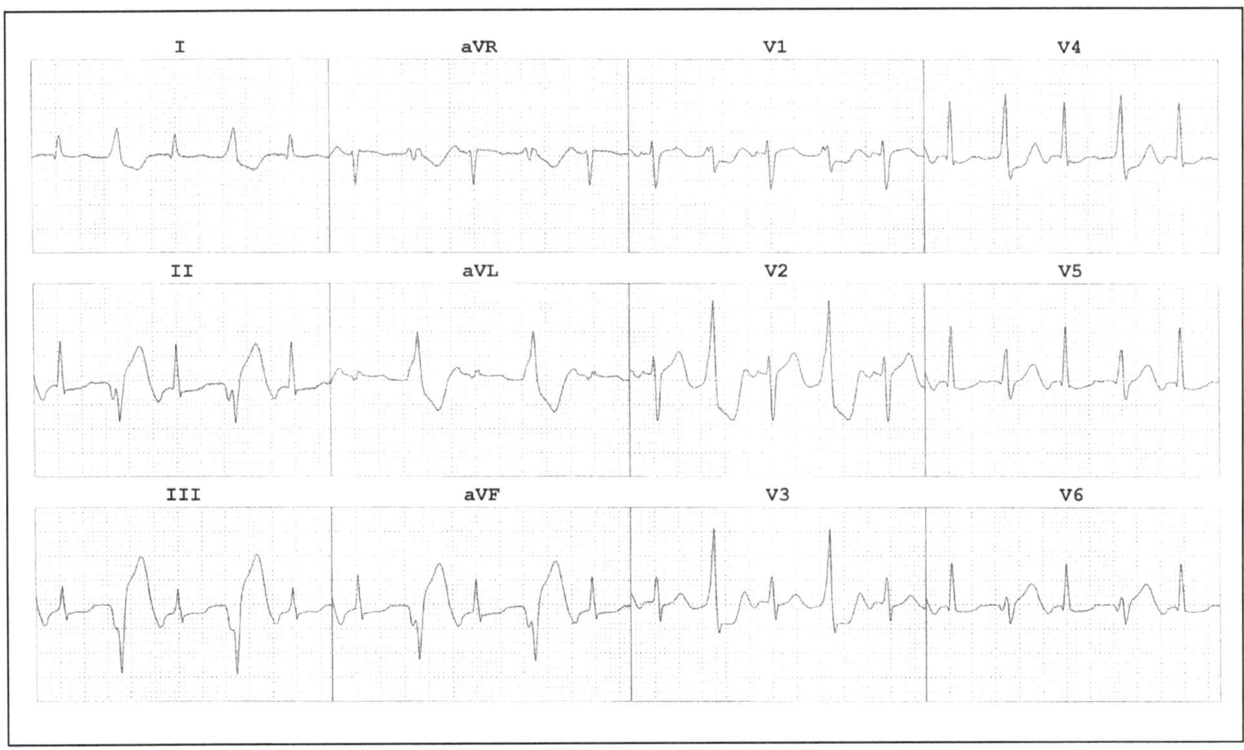

Figure 16.1   A 12-lead ECG of the patient's PVCs.

The PVC originates from the epicardium of the inferobasal septum, also called the "crux of the heart." Clues to the epicardial origin include the sloped onset of the QRS (pseudo-delta wave) that is particularly visible in the inferior and the precordial leads. There is a broad QRS in lead V_1 with a negative terminal deflection. This pattern suggests a left-sided, midline, possibly septal origin. The predominant R wave in the precordial leads suggests a basal origin. In the presence of an inferior axis the origin would likely have been from the aortic cusp. In the presence of a SA, it is from the basal inferior septum. The pseudo-delta wave supports an epicardial origin. In the absence of scarring in the MRI, the presence of Q waves in the inferior leads further argues for an epicardial origin. In this patient, mapping was performed from both the RV and LV septum. The

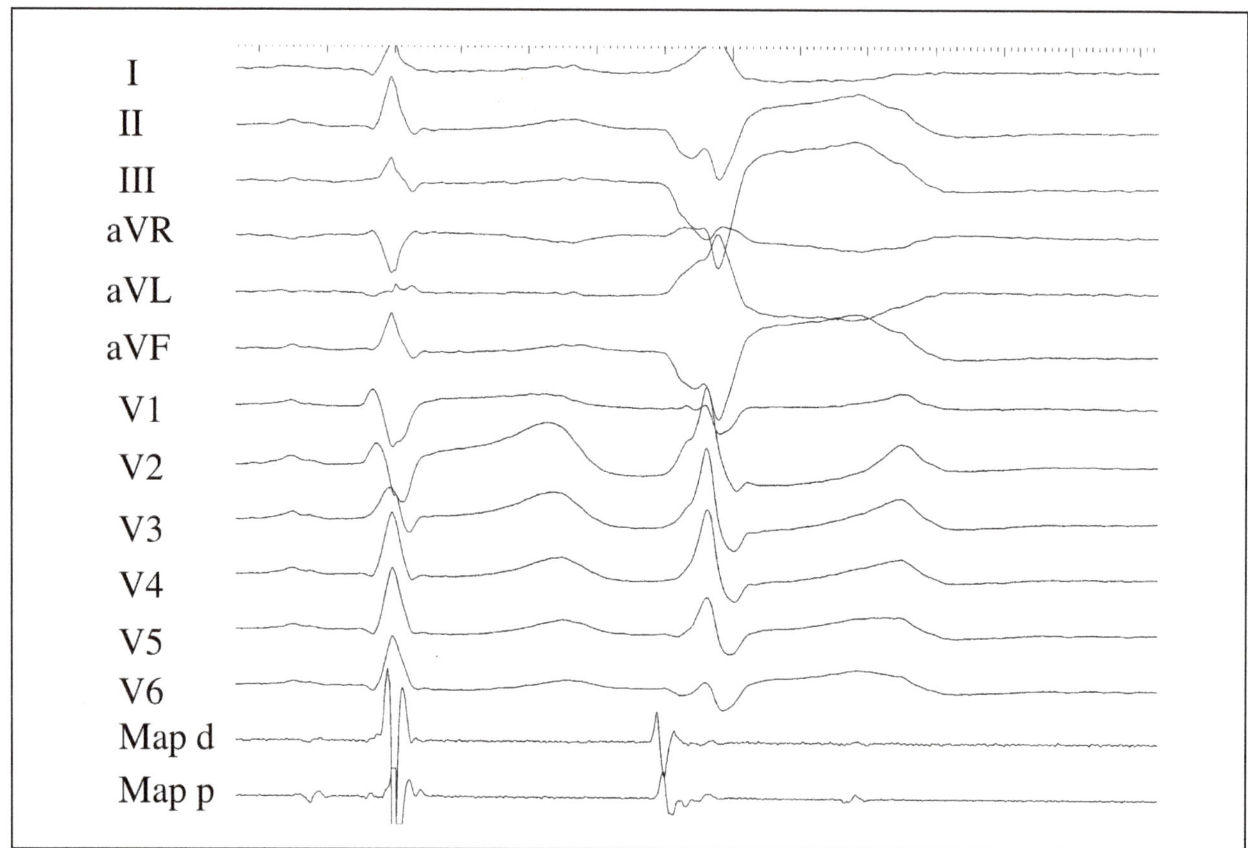

Figure 16.2 Intracardiac tracings with the mapping catheter located in the middle cardiac vein. There is early timing recorded in the distal poles of the mapping catheter (**Map d**) with an activation time of −35 ms.

timing at the inferior RV septum was −20 ms without a matching pace map, and RF ablation failed to eliminate the PVC. The same was observed at the RV septum, where ablation failed. While repeat mapping of the RV was performed, the catheter recorded the earliest electrogram so far: −35 ms (**Figure 16.2**). Initially, it was not clear where the catheter was located until contrast was injected through the irrigation port of the irrigated-tip ablation catheter (**Figure 16.3**). It was thereby determined that the catheter was in the middle cardiac vein. After injection of the coronary arteries documented a safe distance from the posterior descending artery, RF energy was delivered and it eliminated the PVC. **Figure 16.4** displays an activation map of RV, LV, and the middle cardiac vein.

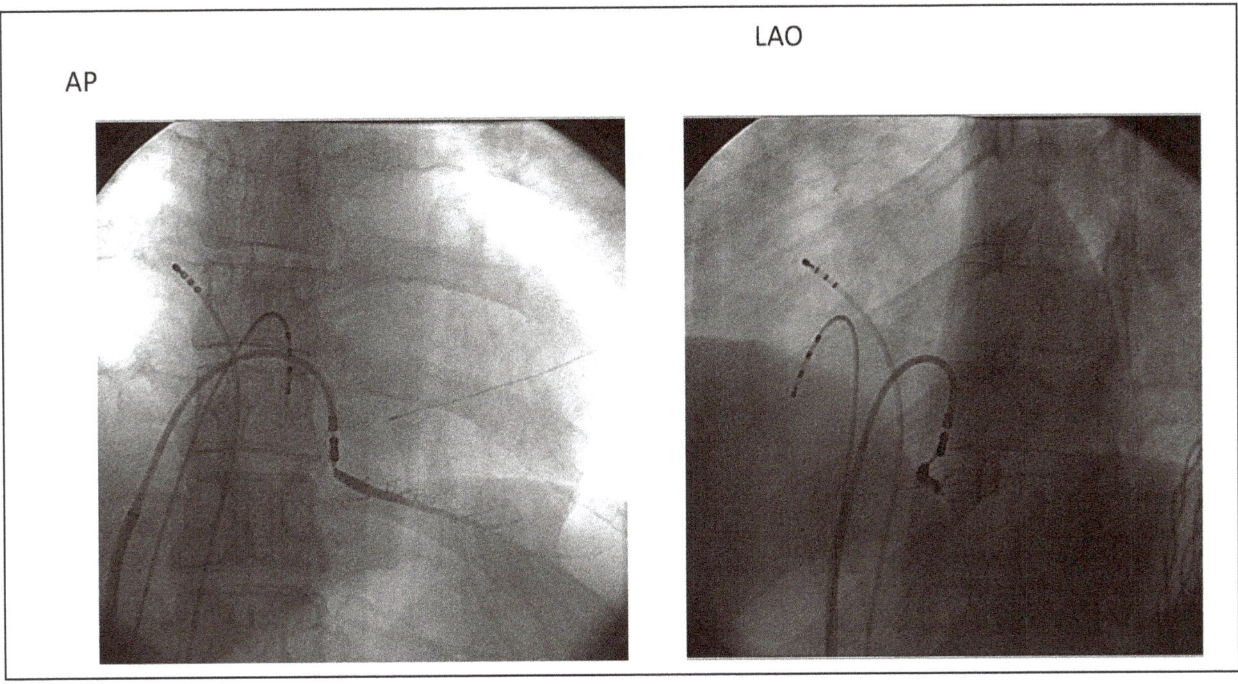

Figure 16.3 **Left panel:** Anteroposterior (AP) view with injection of contrast via the irrigated tip catheter, demonstrating that it is located in the middle cardiac vein. **Right panel:** Left anterior oblique (LAO) view during contrast injection.

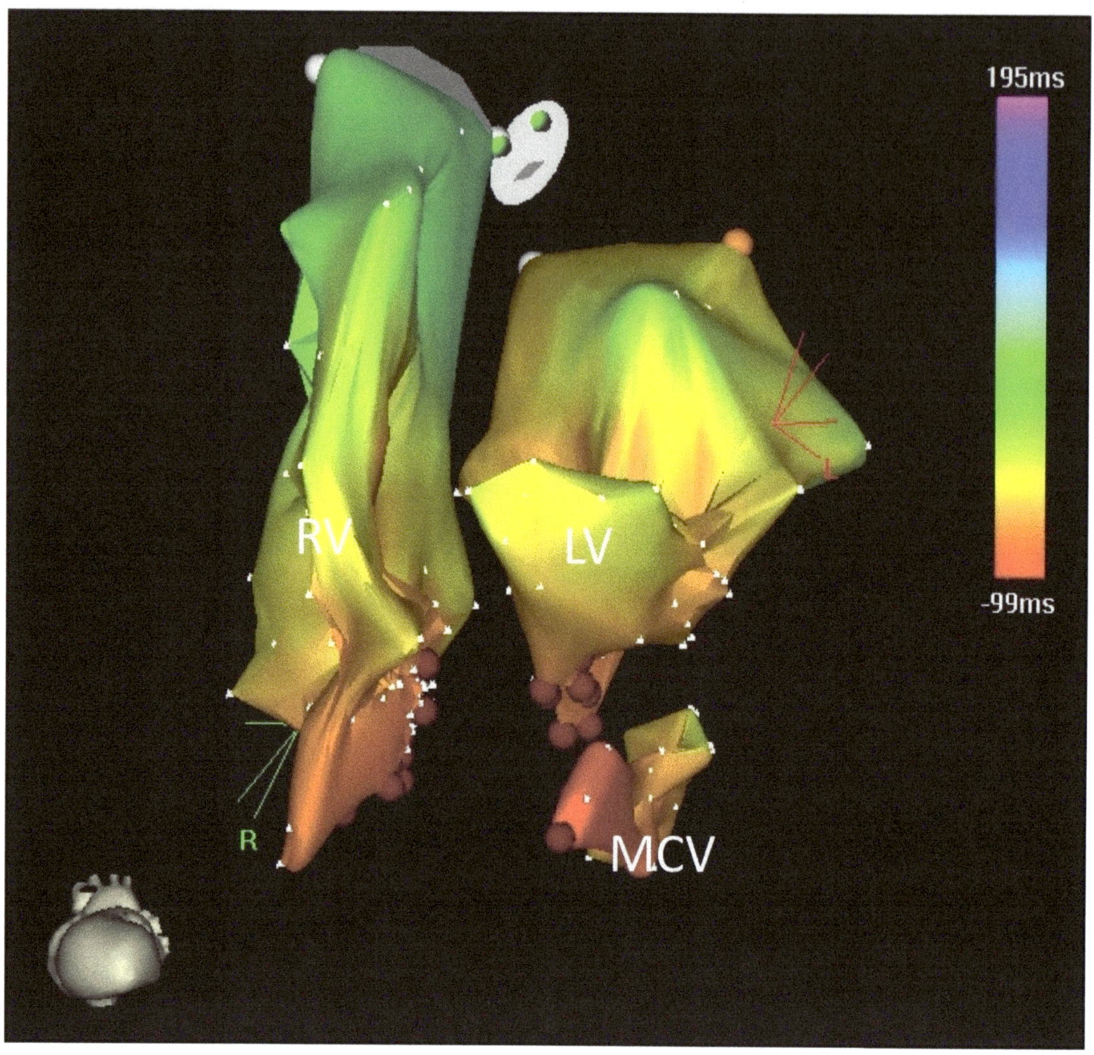

Figure 16.4 Activation map of the left and right ventricles (LV and RV) and the middle cardiac vein (MCV).

CLINICAL HISTORY

A 36-year-old woman, who has had a history of palpitations for 20 years, has experienced worsening of her condition over the past two years. Palpitations were associated with the documented arrhythmia in **Figure 17.1**. She has a structurally normal heart based on echocardiography, stress testing, and cardiac MRI. Two years earlier, an attempted ablation at the distal RV septum that was performed at an outside institution was unsuccessful. Palpitations improved somewhat with calcium-channel blocker therapy, but since her ablation, she has experienced five episodes of syncope, with the last episode occurring only a few weeks prior to her hospital admission. On admission, she reported having palpitations and presyncope several times a week. The patient was referred for an ablation procedure.

Question

Where is the origin of the VT located?

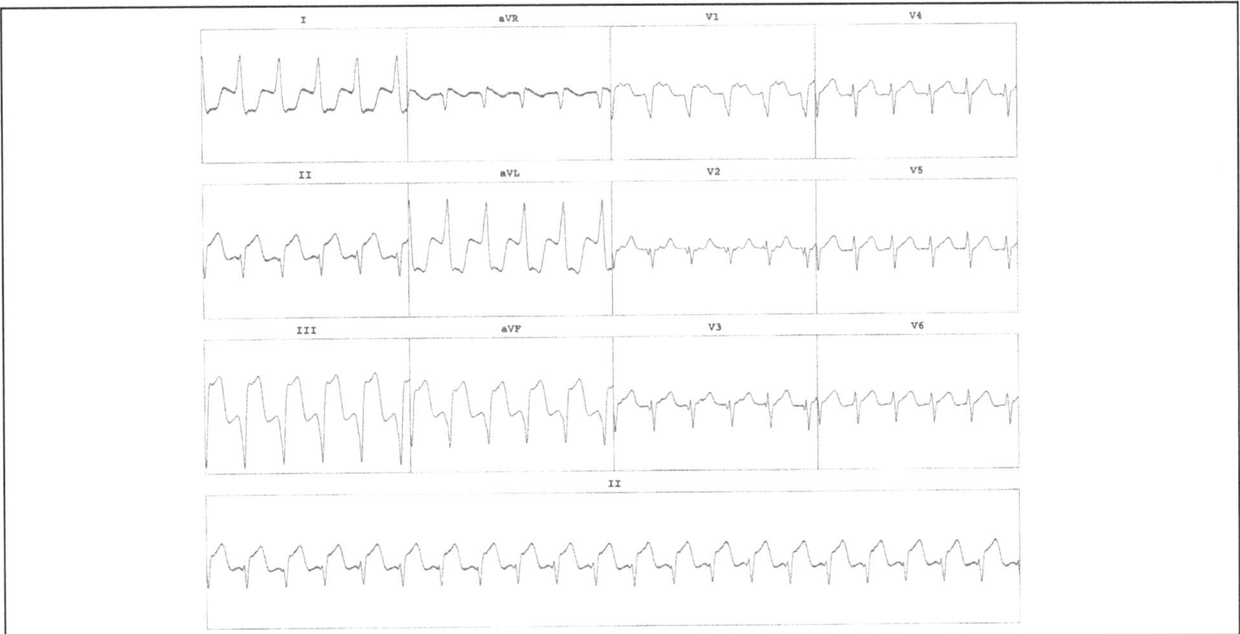

Figure 17.1   A 12-lead ECG of the patient's VT.

Answer

The origin of the VT was intramural with an exit closer to the LV septum than the RV septum. We were unable to identify a matching pace map of this VT with mapping from the LV and RV (**Figure 17.2** and **Figure 17.3** show the best pace map from the site of earliest activation and the location of the pace maps). The earliest timing was on the LV septum (Figure 17.2 and Figure 17.3). The septum had a thickness of 1.5 cm (**Figure 17.4**). The QRS morphology does not suggest a fascicular origin, but the QRS width is quite narrow at 130 ms, which suggests that the conduction system is invaded by the VT focus. The slope of the initial part of the QRS is slow especially in the inferior leads but encounters a more rapid deflection later in the QRS (leads II, V_2–V_5).

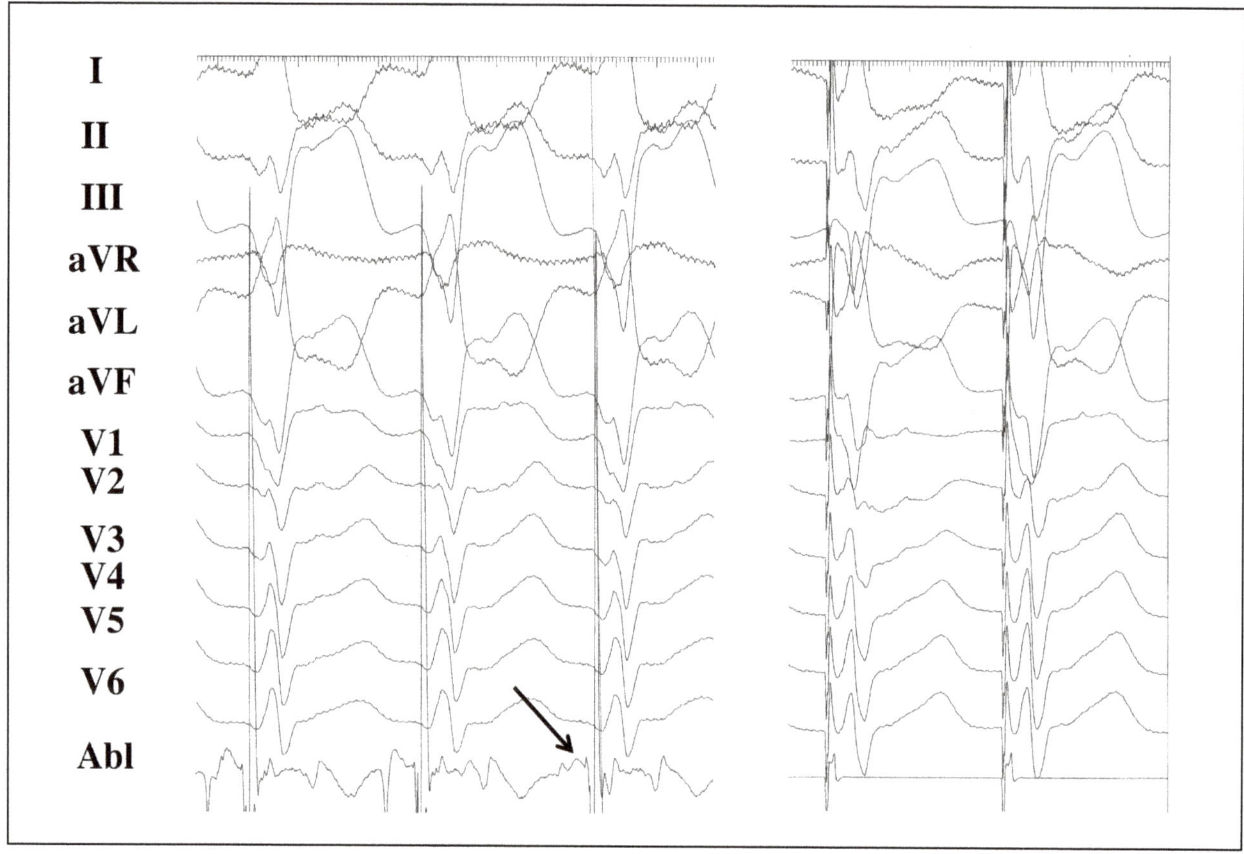

Figure 17.2 **Left panel:** VT at the site of earliest left ventricular endocardial activation (**arrow**). **Right panel:** Pace map at this site shows a similar but different QRS morphology that did not match the VT QRS morphology.

The patient was referred for ablation of a suspected fascicular VT. The morphology of a fascicular VT, however, is a typical RBBB morphology with an rsR′ morphology in V_1 and a left- or right-axis morphology depending on the origin from the posterior or the anterior fascicle, respectively. There are often small q waves in the lateral limb leads I and aVL for posterior fascicular VTs. During the mapping procedure, sites with Purkinje potentials were sought during sinus rhythm, but they did not precede the QRS complex during VT. Mapping focused on the earliest endocardial activation of both RV and LV septum. RF energy was delivered at both RV and LV septum (Figure 17.3). The effective lesion was on the LV septum at a site with a poor pace map, without Purkinje potentials, and an activation time of −22 ms (Figure 17.2).

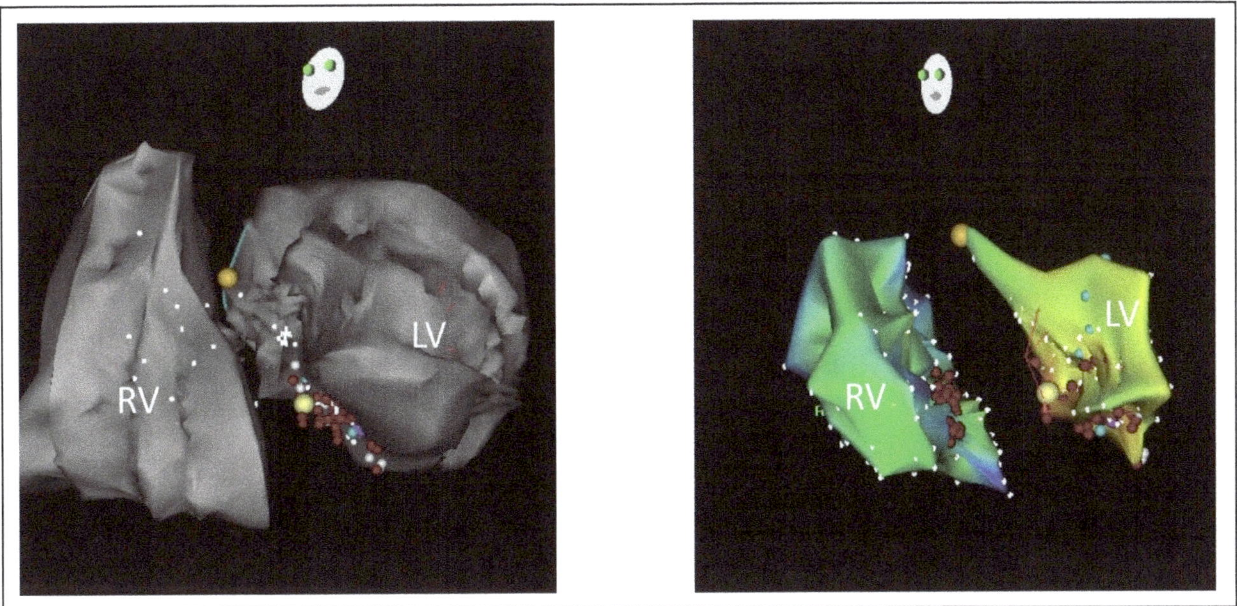

Figure 17.3 **Left panel:** 3D reconstruction of both right and left ventricles (RV and LV). **Right panel:** Activation maps obtained during VT. The successful ablation site is indicated with a **yellow tag**. The His location is shown with a **orange tag**.

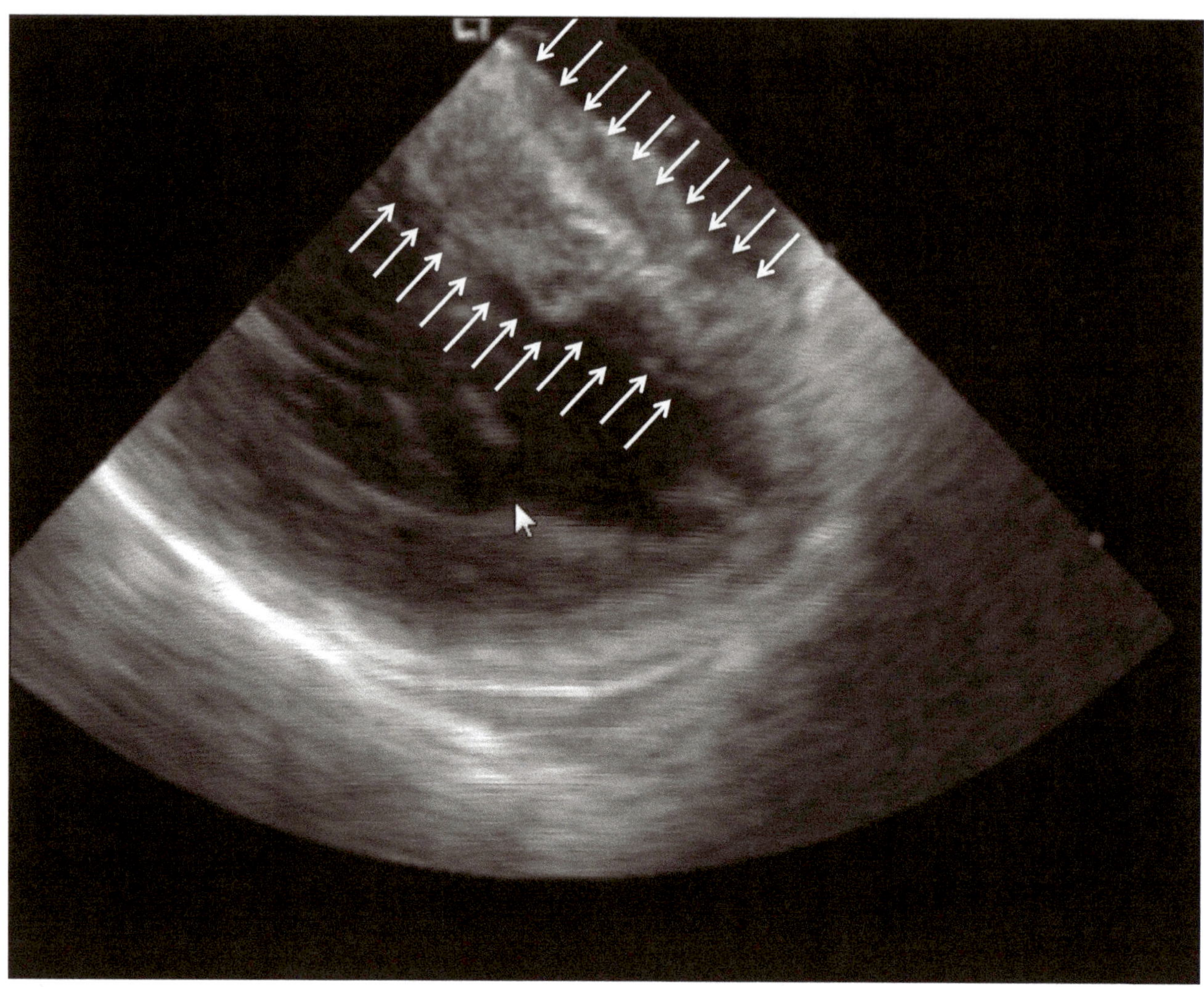

Figure 17.4 The interventricular septum at the site of ablation as seen by intracardiac ultrasound. **Arrows** indicate the septal thickness of 1.5 cm.

CLINICAL HISTORY

A 59-year-old African American woman has had a prior anterior wall myocardial infarction and a failed VT ablation procedure from an outside hospital. Her VT was controlled with amiodarone. The patient, however, wished to stop taking amiodarone. Her ejection fraction was 20% and there was a large anterior wall aneurysm. The patient was referred for a repeat VT ablation procedure.

Question

Where is the exit site of the VT shown in **Figure 18.1**, and what is the mechanism of the findings occurring during pacing in **Figure 18.2**?

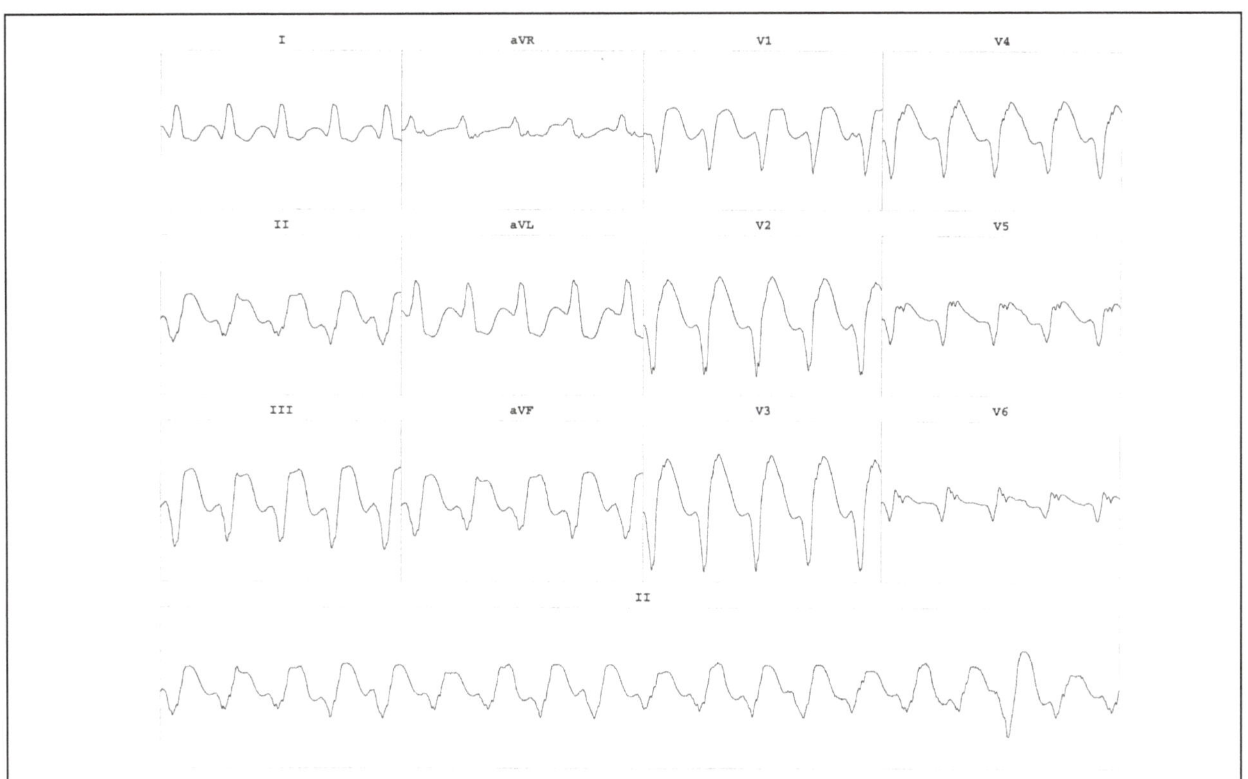

Figure 18.1   A 12-lead ECG of the inducible VT.

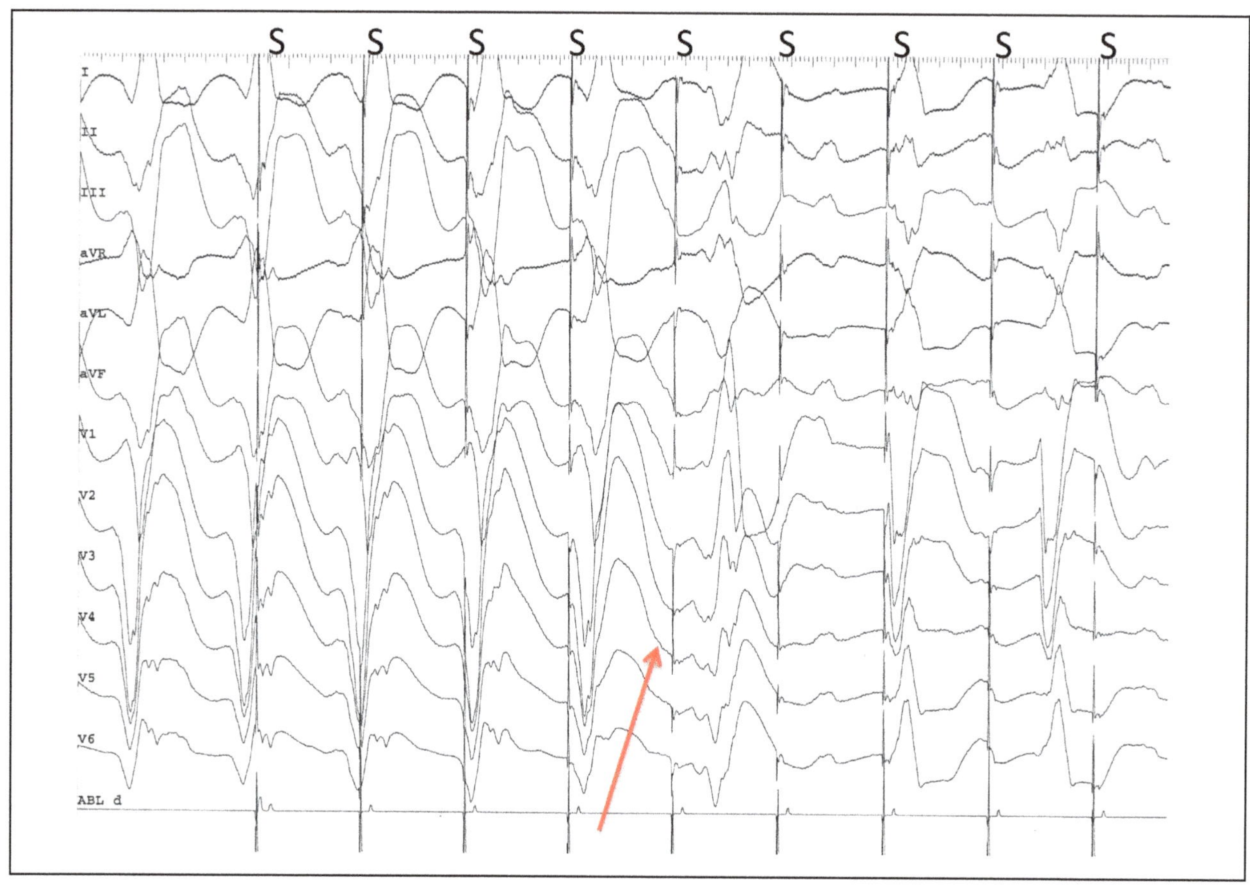

Figure 18.2 A 12-lead ECG and intracardiac electrograms while pacing is performed from the mapping catheter (**S**). VT terminates with a stimulus that does not result in global ventricular capture (**red arrow**).

Answer

During the procedure, only one VT was inducible. This was also the clinical VT. The VT was hemodynamically tolerated and could be mapped. The morphology was a LBBB morphology: i.e., the exit site is expected to be located on the septum, most likely the LV septum. The axis is superior with Q waves in the inferior leads, indicating an origin from the inferior wall, and there is negative concordance, indicating an apical origin. The exit should be the inferoapical septum. However, it is unclear whether the exit is endocardial (LV or RV), epicardial (inferior part of the septum), or intramural. We were not able to get a good match with the VT morphology with a short stimulus-QRS interval and thus were unable to identify the VT exit. Provided the VT is tolerated, it may not be necessary to identify the exit site to eliminate the VT, as long as there is a critical component of the VT circuit that can be reached with the catheter. The patient's VT was hemodynamically tolerated, and in the anterior aspect of the aneurysm, we identified the site shown in Figure 18.2. Figure 18.2 shows VT termination with nonglobal capture when pacing during VT was attempted.[1] This is usually a critical site indicating a narrow isthmus.

Figure 18.3 shows concealed entrainment with a matching stimulus–QRS and electrogram–QRS interval indicating that the catheter is in contact with a critical site of the reentry circuit and radiofrequency energy delivery resulted in permanent VT termination at this site. **Figure 18.4** shows the location this site (arrow). Had the VT not been tolerated, identifying these sites would not have been possible by using pace mapping alone, since the exit site was not reachable from the endocardium. The MRI showed intramural delayed enhancement in the septum, and therefore it is not surprising that we were unable to identify the exit site from the LV or RV endocardium despite extensive pace mapping. This case provides a strong argument not to map/ablate exclusively in the border zone. The sites critical to this VT were in the center of the scar (Figure 18.4) and extensive ablation in the border zone during the prior ablation procedure at the outside hospital failed to eliminate this VT.[2]

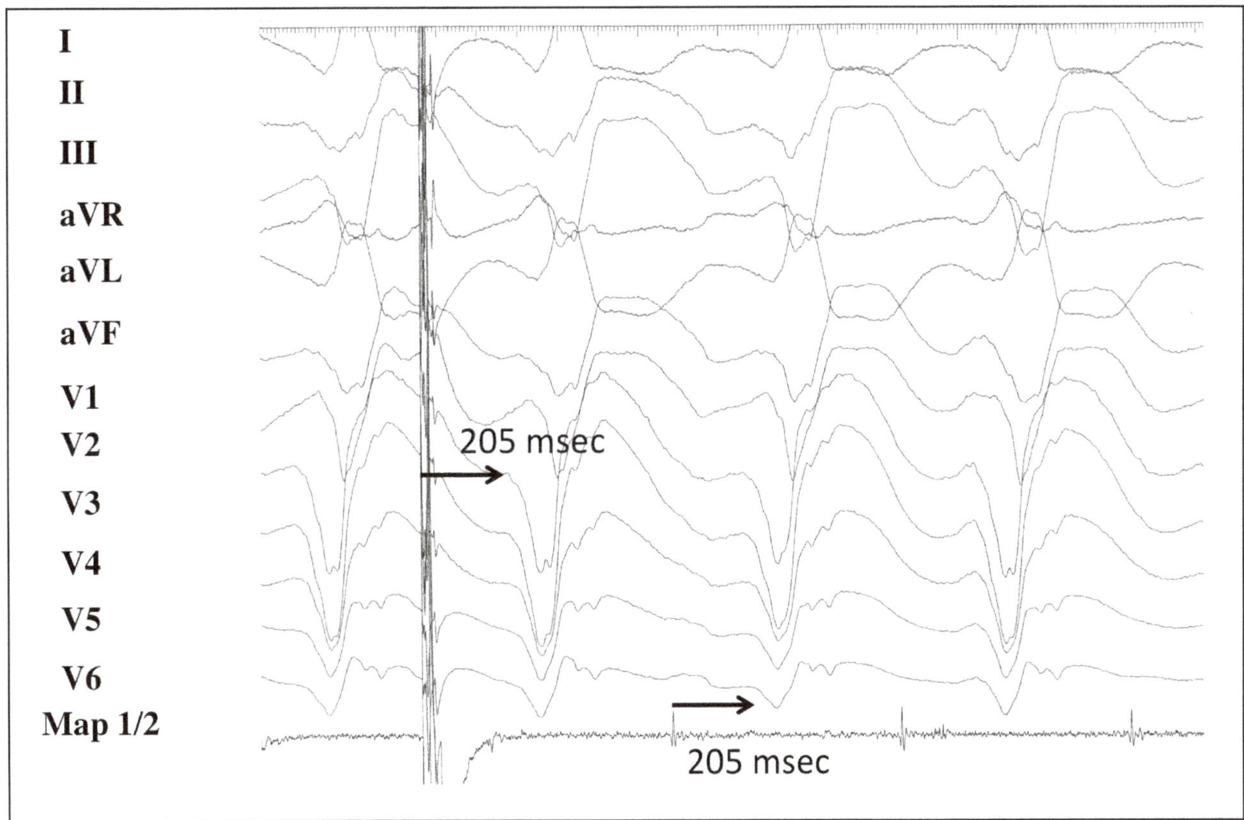

Figure 18.3 This figure shows a site with concealed entrainment. The stimulus-QRS interval is equal to the electrogram-QRS interval (both measure 205 ms). This was the successful ablation site.

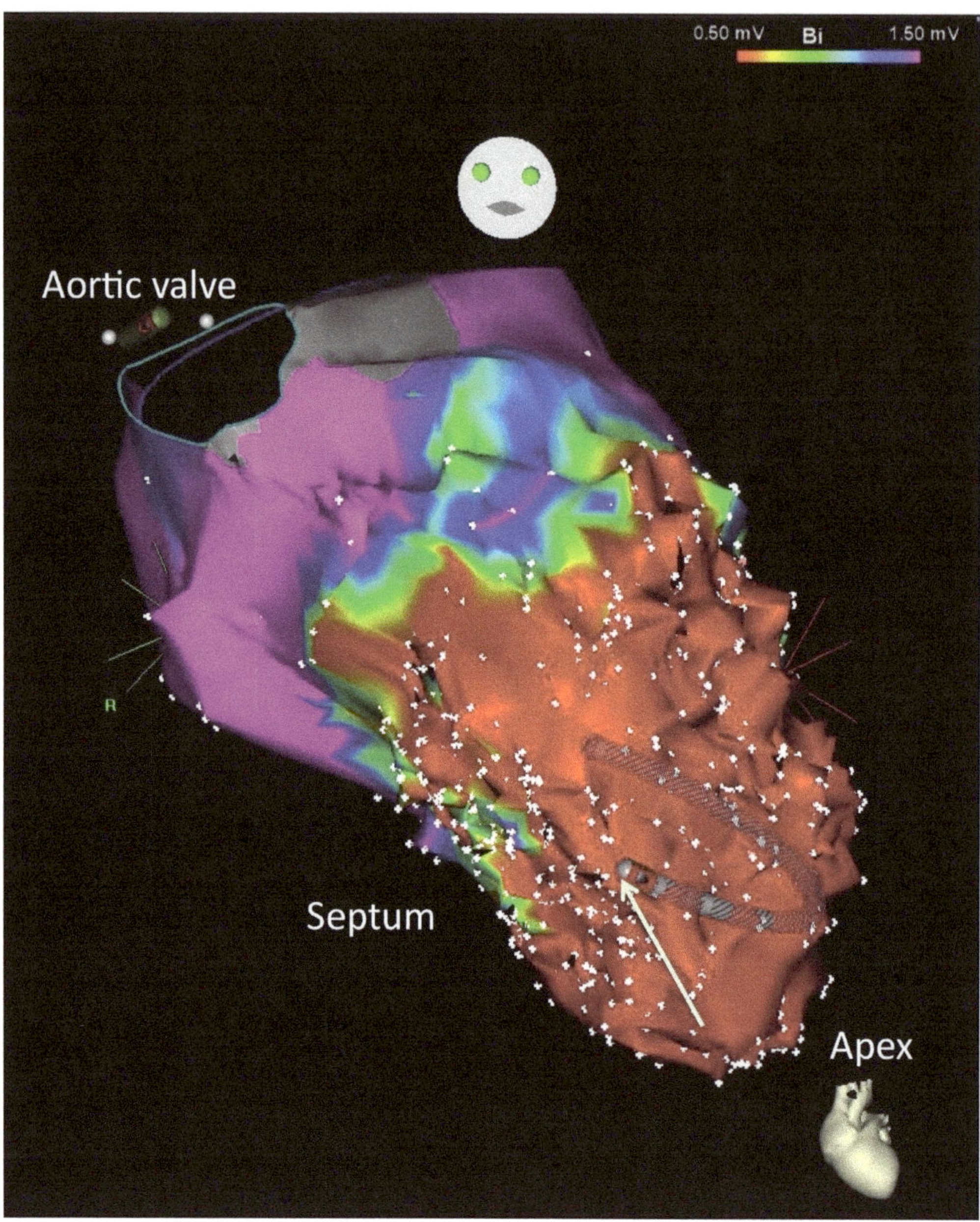

Figure 18.4 Electroanatomic map showing the anterior septal aspect of the left ventricle. A **white arrow** marks the site where nonglobal capture and later concealed entrainment was documented and radiofrequency ablation resulted in elimination of VT.

REFERENCES

1. Bogun F, Krishnan SC, Marine JE, et al. Catheter ablation guided by termination of post-infarction ventricular tachycardia by pacing with non-global capture. *Heart Rhythm.* 2004;1:422–426.
2. Sinno MC, Yokokawa M, Good E, et al. Endocardial ablation of postinfarction ventricular tachycardia with nonendocardial exit sites. *Heart Rhythm.* 2013;10:794–799.

CLINICAL HISTORY

A 47-year-old woman presented with a history of symptomatic PVCs, resulting in palpitations, chest pain, dizziness, and lightheadedness. There was no history of syncope and no family history of sudden cardiac death. A Holter monitor showed frequent PVCs (PVC 12,000 beats/48 hours), and there were late potentials on the signal-averaged ECG. Her echocardiogram showed normal right and left ventricular sizes and function. There were no wall motion abnormalities or delayed enhancement on cardiac MRI.

Question

Where do the PVCs shown in **Figure 19.1** originate?

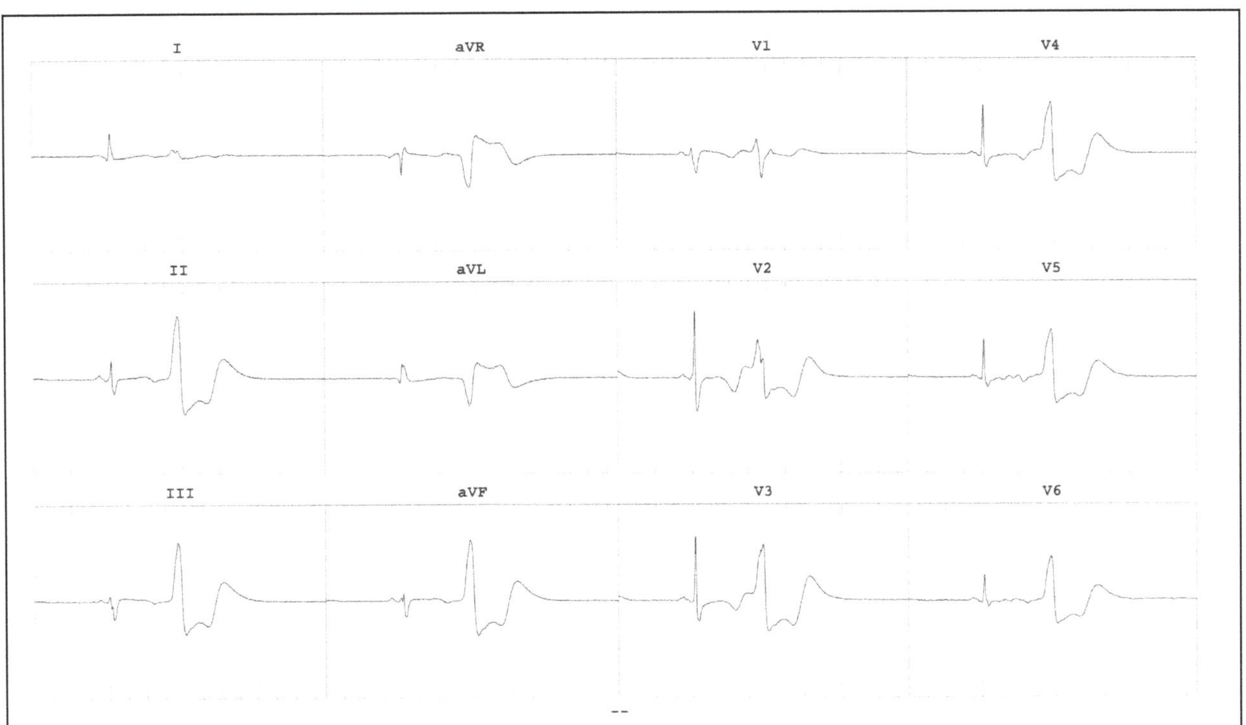

Figure 19.1   A 12-lead ECG of the patient's PVC.

Answer

The origin was located intramurally between the posterior RVOT and the right/left commissure of the aortic cusp. The broad R wave and the early transition point towards an origin in the aortic cusps (Figure 19.1).[1] Mapping in the RVOT, however, showed early timing of −30 ms (**Figure 19.2**) and pace maps that closely matched the target PVC morphology (**Figure 19.3**). In the aortic cusps the timing was later (−21 ms) and the PMs were close, but not as good as in the RVOT (Figure 19.3). RF energy delivery in the RVOT resulted in suppression of the PVCs for some time and recurrence of the PVCs after ~45 minutes. Only after RF energy was delivered in the right coronary cusp (RCC) did the PVCs disappear permanently. No ECG criteria indicating an intramural origin had been described yet. The approximate anatomic origin was indicated by the LBBB (possibly RVOT), inferior axis (outflow tract vs. supravalvular structures), and early transition (< V_3) indicating the possibility of a left-sided origin.[2] In the referenced manuscript by Tanner et al., the majority of patients with early transition had successful ablations in the RVOT. A positive QRS-complex in lead I and the amplitude of lead II > lead III indicate a posterior origin (posterior RVOT or aortic cusps) because the anterior RVOT is oriented more leftward compared to the posterior RVOT that was more rightward oriented.[3]

The extent of T-wave inversions of the sinus rhythm QRS complex across the precordium is a major criterion for ARVC/D and is important to recognize. Based on the 12-lead ECG, the Holter information, and the abnormal signal-averaged ECG, the patient met Task Force Criteria for ARVC/D.[4]

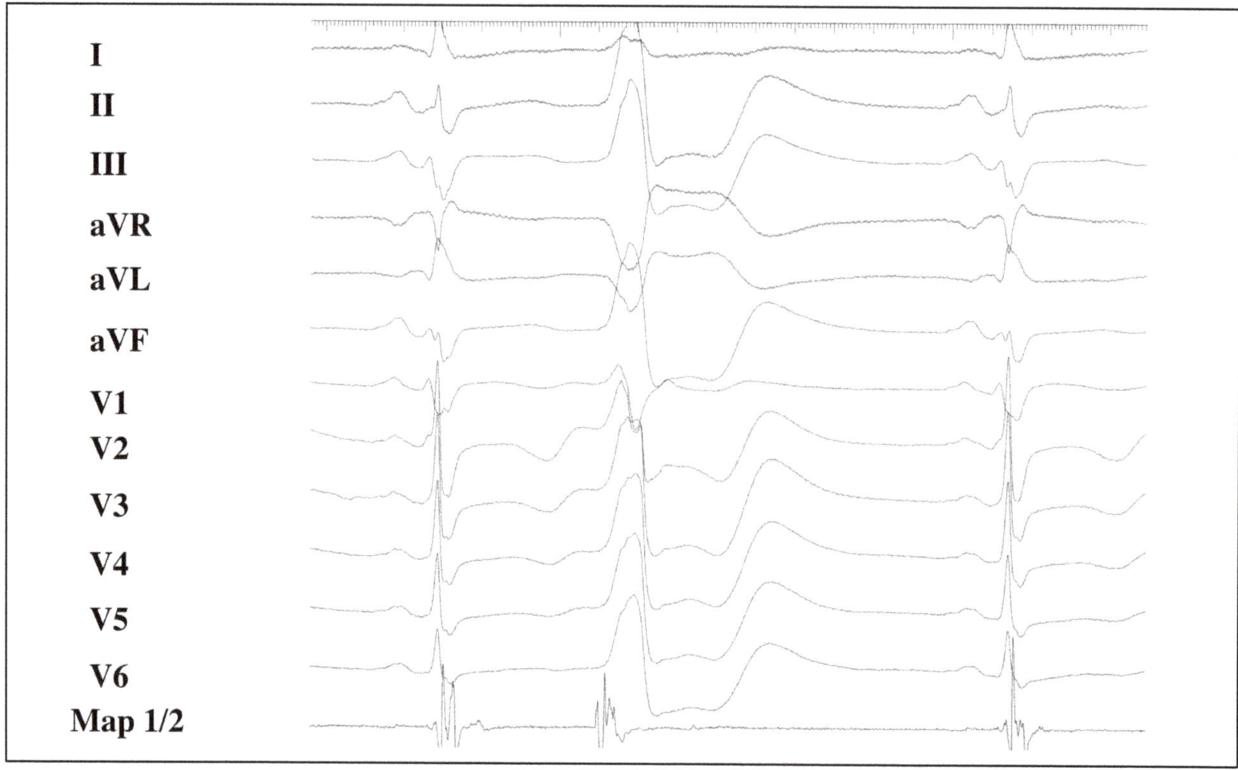

Figure 19.2 Activation map indicating early timing of −30 ms in the RVOT (map 1/2).

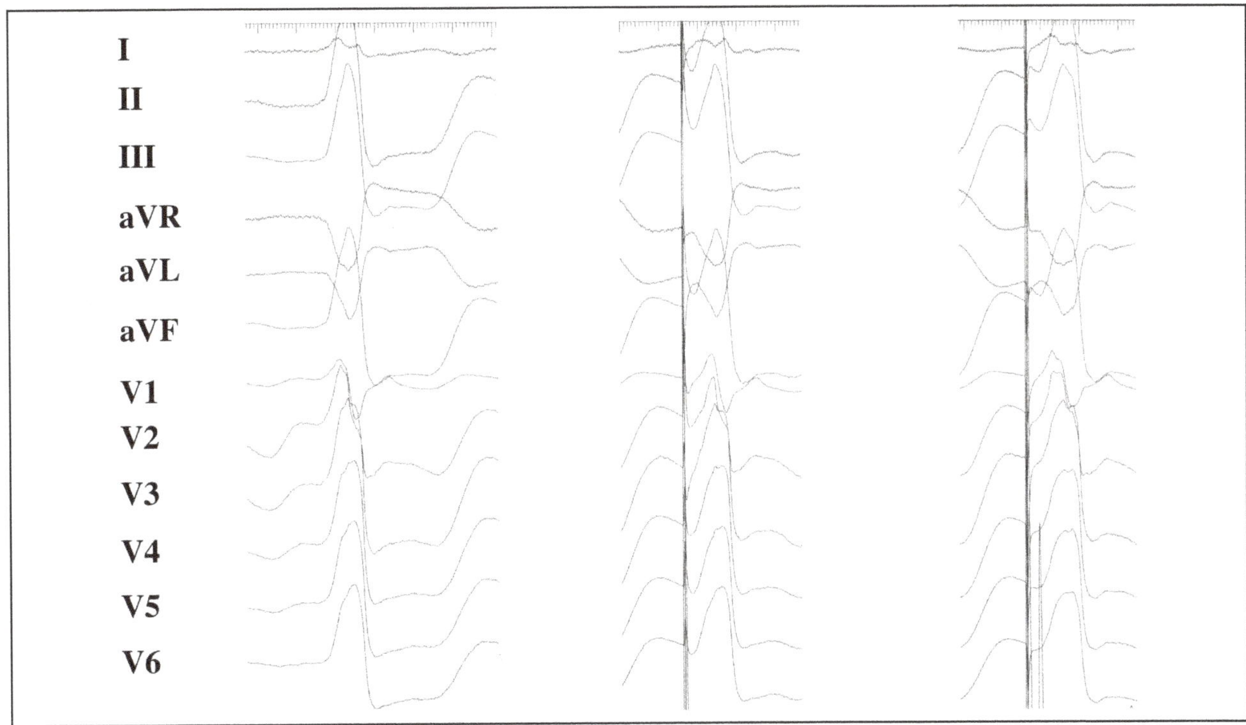

Figure 19.3 **Left panel:** Spontaneous PVC. **Middle panel:** Pace map from the posterior RVOT. **Right panel:** Pace map from the right coronary cusp.

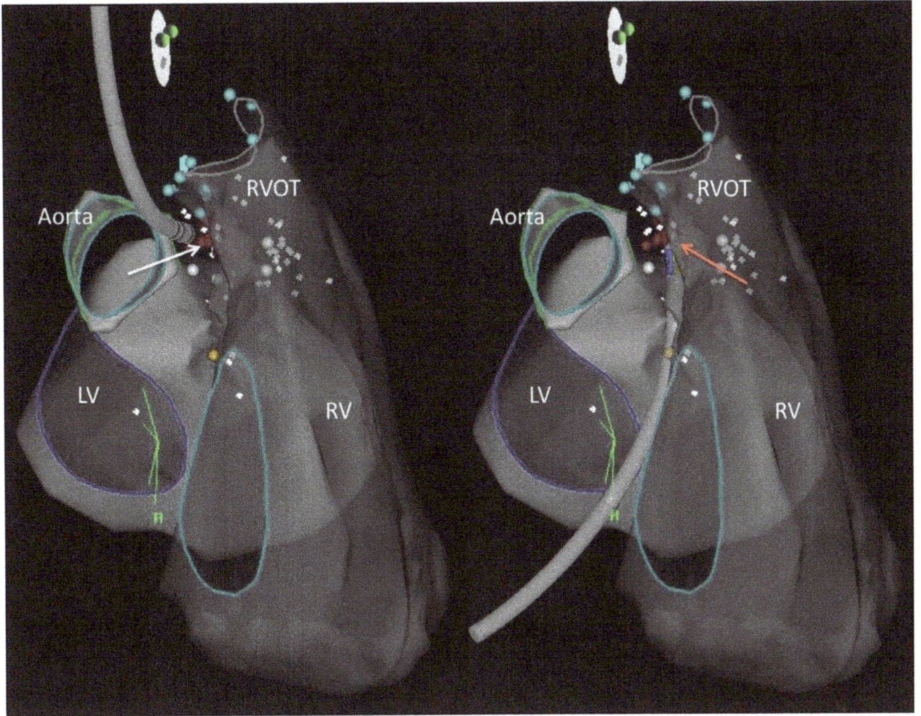

Figure 19.4 3D reconstruction of echocardiographic contours of the left and the right ventricles (LV and RV). **Left panel:** Catheter position in the right coronary cusp (**white arrow**). **Right panel:** Catheter position in the RVOT (**red arrow**). **Light blue tags** indicate the level of the pulmonic valve.

REFERENCES

1. Ouyang F, Fotuhi P, Ho SY, et al. Repetitive monomorphic ventricular tachycardia originating from the aortic sinus cusp: Electrocardiographic characterization for guiding catheter ablation. *J Am Coll Cardiol.* 2002;39:500–508.
2. Tanner H, Hindricks G, Schirdewahn P, et al. Outflow tract tachycardia with r/s transition in lead v3: Six different anatomic approaches for successful ablation. *J Am Coll Cardiol.* 2005;45:418–423.
3. Dixit S, Gerstenfeld EP, Callans DJ, Marchlinski FE. Electrocardiographic patterns of superior right ventricular outflow tract tachycardias: Distinguishing septal and free-wall sites of origin. *J Cardiovasc Electrophysiol.* 2003;14:1–7.
4. Marcus FI, McKenna WJ, Sherrill D, et al. Diagnosis of arrhythmogenic right ventricular cardiomyopathy/dysplasia: Proposed modification of the task force criteria. *Circulation.* 2010;121:1533–1541.

CLINICAL HISTORY

A 74-year-old man presented with a history of hypertension, hyperlipidemia, and diabetes, as well as frequent PVCs for several years. He was mostly asymptomatic other than being fatigued most of the time. His PVC burden has been as high as 24% by Holter monitoring, and his most recent echocardiogram showed an ejection fraction of 25%. A cardiac catheterization showed no occlusive coronary artery disease.

He was in NYHA functional class II. His cardiac MRI showed a mildly dilated left ventricle with mild to moderately reduced left ventricular systolic function of 41%. Left ventricular ejection fraction was 41%. Nonspecific mid-myocardial delayed enhancement within the left ventricle compatible with dilated cardiomyopathy was also noted.

Question

Where does the PVC in **Figure 20.1** originate, and how should it be targeted?

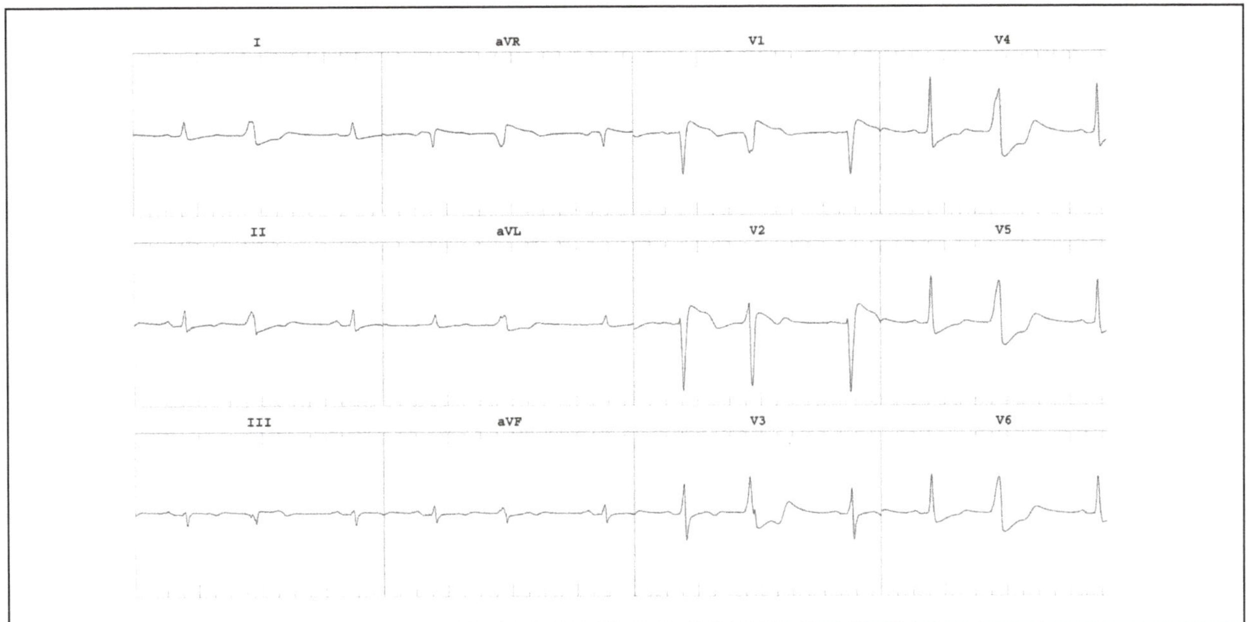

Figure 20.1   A 12-lead ECG of the predominant PVC.

This patient has an intramural origin that corresponded to the intramural scar located in the high septum. The site was about 1 cm below the location of the His bundle. Characteristics for a site close to the His bundle include the following: 1) LBBB with a QS pattern in V_1; 2) large R-wave amplitude in lead I that is greater than the R wave in any of the inferior leads; 3) positive R wave in lead aVL.[1] The observation that lead II is more positive than lead III indicates a more posterior origin in the RV as compared to the anterior RV and RVOT. Furthermore, on the level of the atrioventricular valves, the RV is oriented towards the right, whereas the RVOT is located more toward the left. This explains the positive R wave in leads I and aVL, as well as, the discrepancy of leads II being positive (more rightward of the tricuspid valve area) and lead III being negative (vector

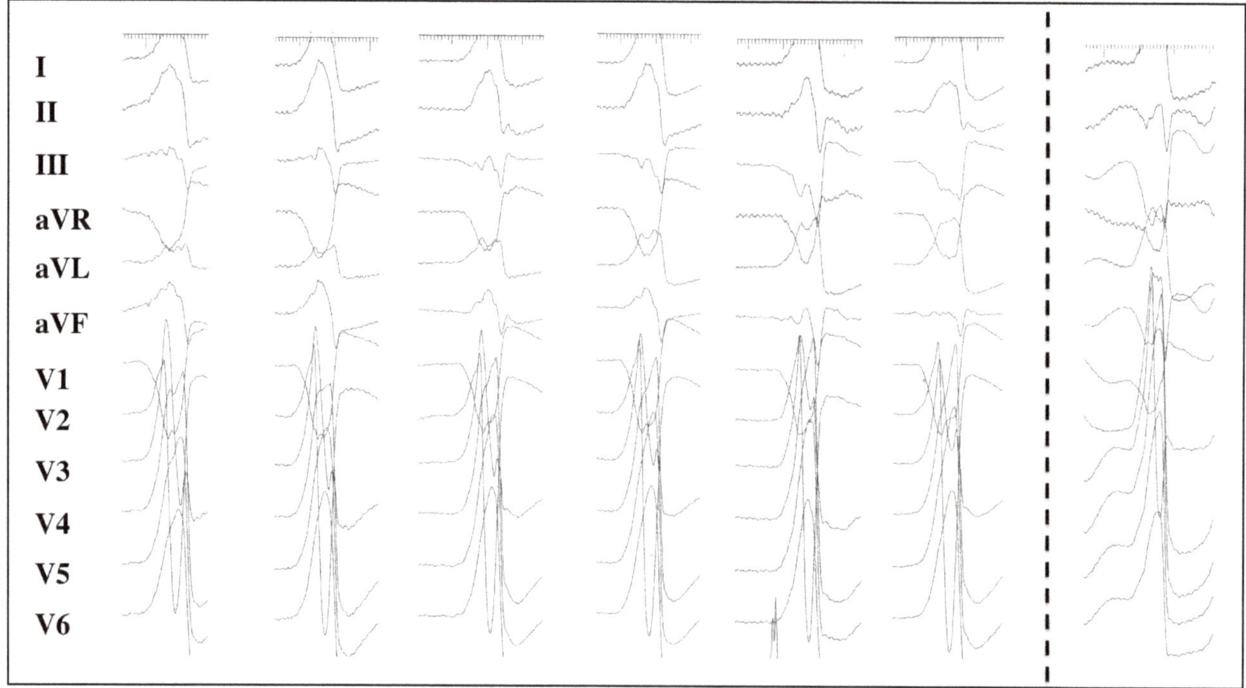

Figure 20.2 This figure shows spontaneously occurring PVCs with different morphologies prior to ablation (**to the left of the dashed line**) and after ablation targeting an endocardial breakthrough site close to the His bundle (**right to dashed line**).

going towards the left, i.e., away from lead III). **Figure 20.2** shows the spectrum of the spontaneous variations observed from the intramural PVC. All of them have the features of a parahisian origin. **Figure 20.3** shows a target site where activation was early (–35 ms). However, the pace map did not match, which is typical for intramural origins.

RF energy was delivered at this location since it was at a safe distance from the conduction system. Thereafter, the PVC morphology changed its axis (**Figure 20.4**), becoming negative in all inferior leads. This new PVC morphology was also targeted and thereafter, PVCs did not recur. The change in morphology is not unusual when breakout sites of intramural arrhythmias are targeted.

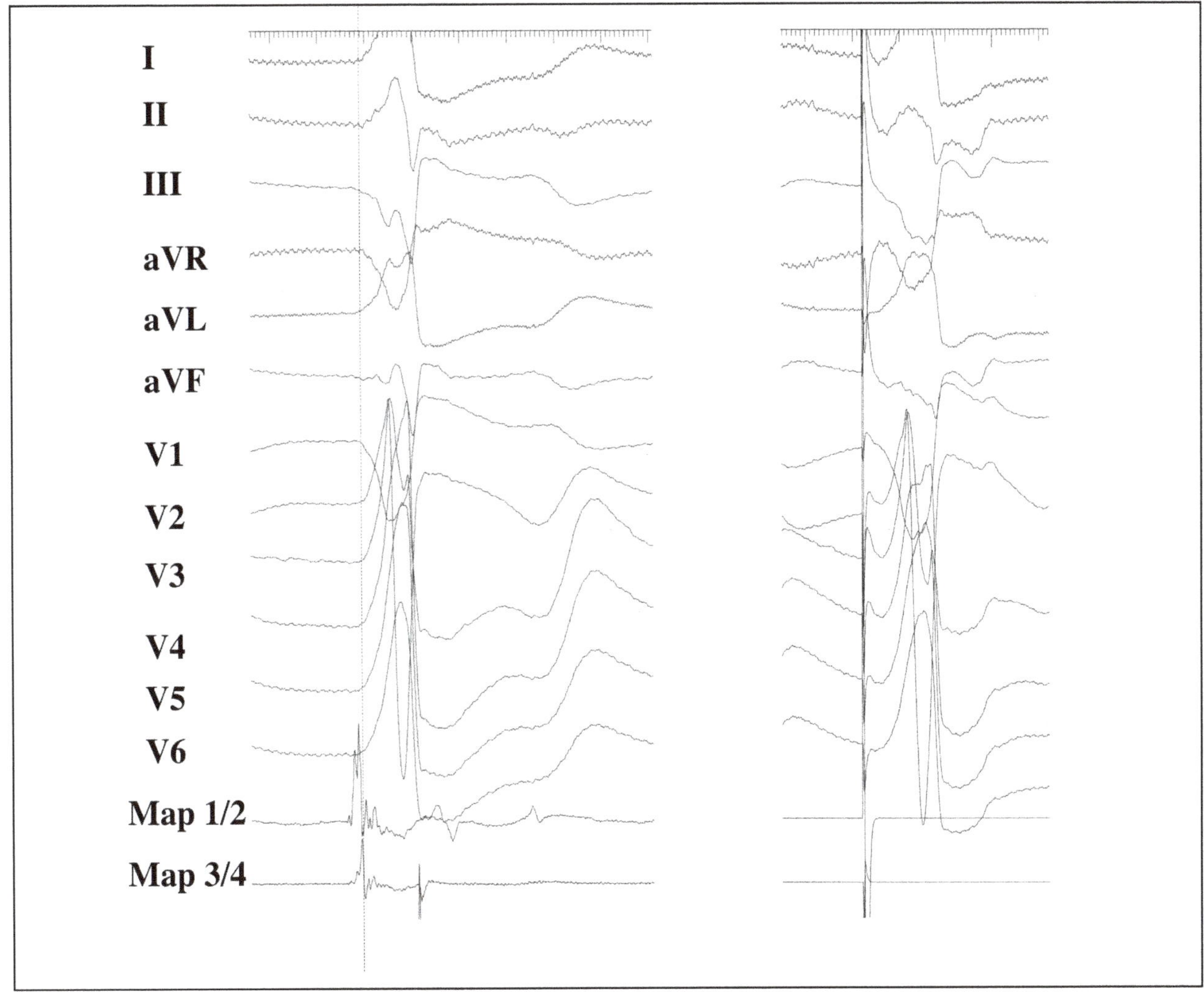

Figure 20.3　**Left panel:** Activation time of the PVC at the endocardial breakout site (–35 ms). **Right panel:** Pace map at this site failed to show a matching pace map.

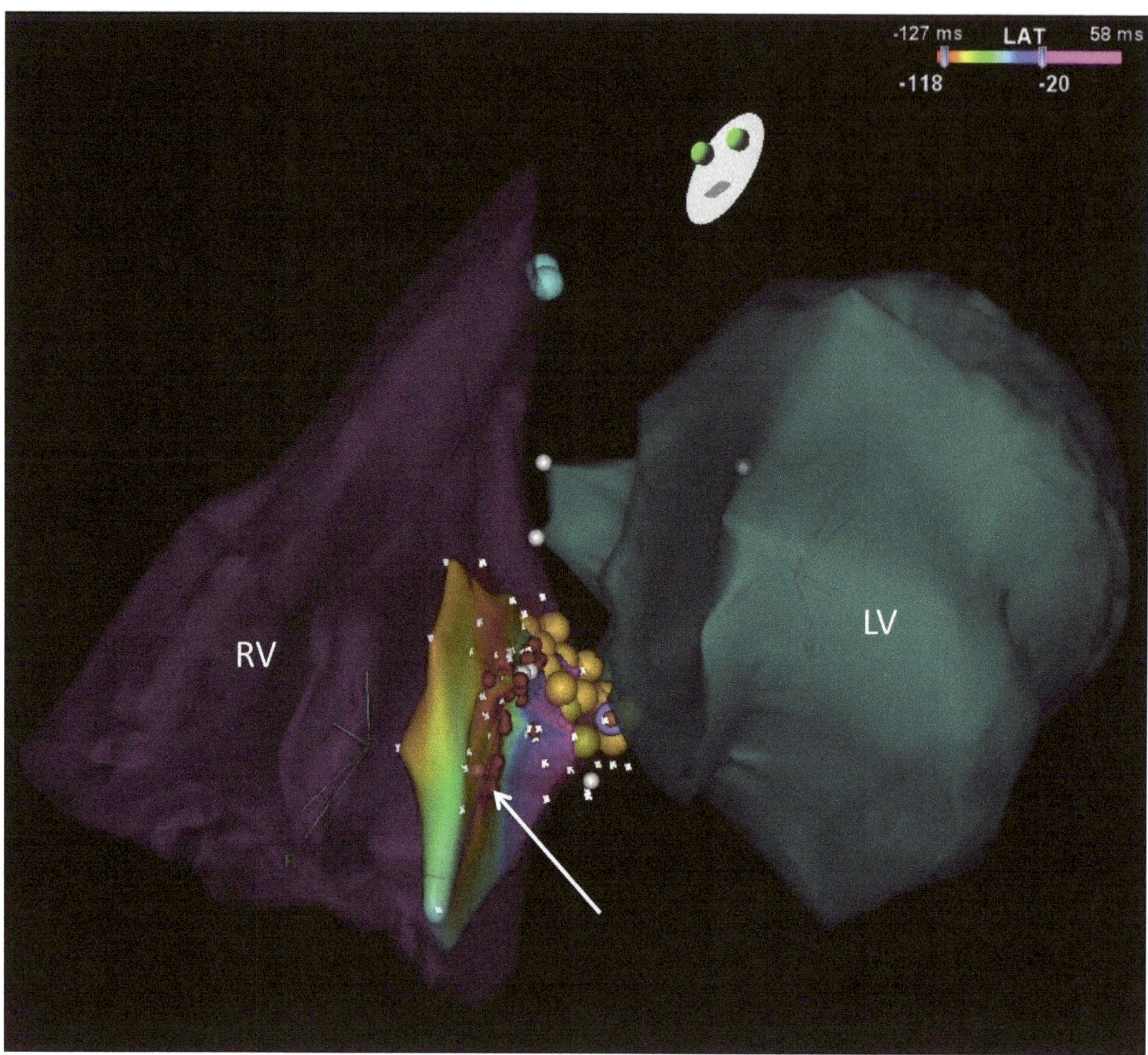

Figure 20.4   3D echocardiographic reconstruction of left and right ventricles (RV and LV) with **orange tags** indicating the location of a His cloud and red tags indicating ablation lesions. The **white arrows** indicate where the final targeted PVC was breaking out and where RF energy was applied.

The transition in the parahisian area can be early or late. An earlier transition, however, does not necessarily indicate a left-sided origin. In this patient, activation mapping in the aortic cusp and the LVOT did not show in any of the early sites.

REFERENCE

1. Yamauchi Y, Aonuma K, Takahashi A, et al. Electrocardiographic characteristics of repetitive monomorphic right ventricular tachycardia originating near the his-bundle. *J Cardiovasc Electrophysiol.* 2005;16:1041–1048.

CLINICAL HISTORY

The patient from Case 20 had another PVC morphology (**Figure 21.1**) that was frequent and was also mapped.

Question

Where did this PVC originate from, and based on the information provided in **Figure 21.2**, is this a good ablation site?

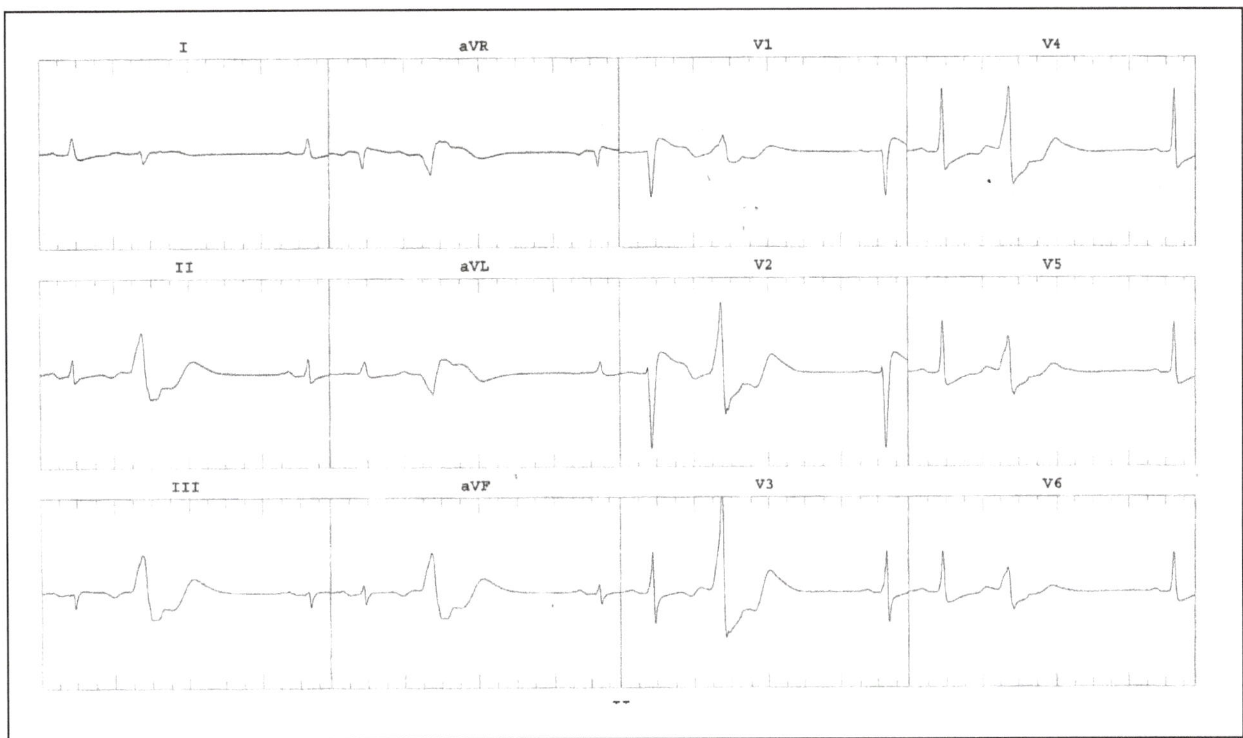

Figure 21.1   A 12-lead ECG of the patient's PVC.

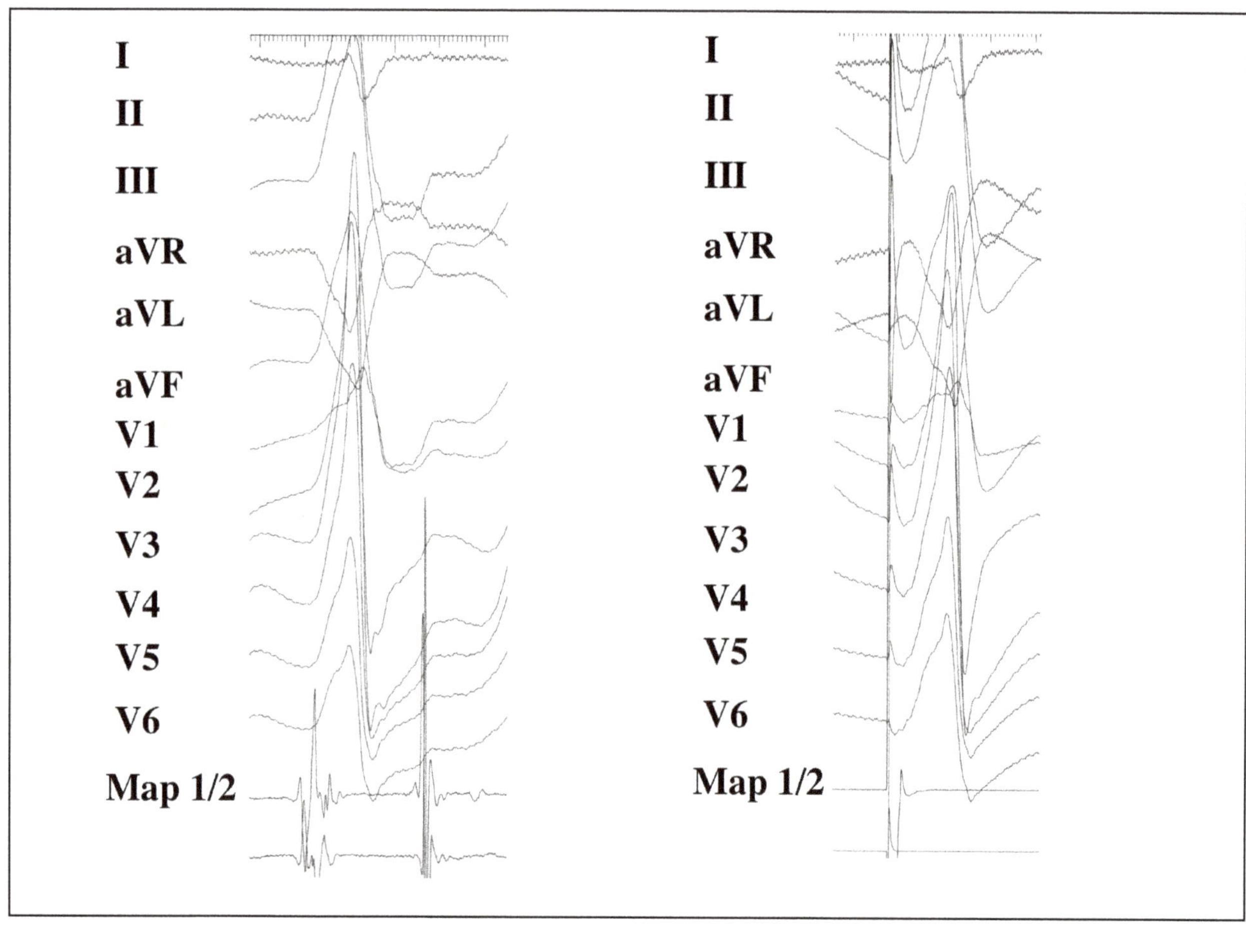

Figure 21.2 **Left panel:** Activation map of the PVC showing an activation time of –30 ms within the distal great cardiac vein. **Right panel:** Pace map at this location showing a matching pace map with the spontaneous PVC.

Answer

This PVC originated from the basal, anterior, LV epicardium (**Figure 21.3**). The hints for this location are the following features: inferior axis (i.e., anterior location in the LV), positive concordance across the precordium (indicating a basal origin), decreased initial slope in lead V_1 (pseudo–delta wave), as well as isoelectric to negative QRS in lead I (i.e., lead I does not start with an r wave; this supports an epicardial origin). Based on the mapping data shown in Figure 21.2, i.e., early timing and matching pace map, this would be a great site for an ablation. However, one also needs to make sure that the catheter within the coronary venous system (CVS) is not too close to a coronary artery.

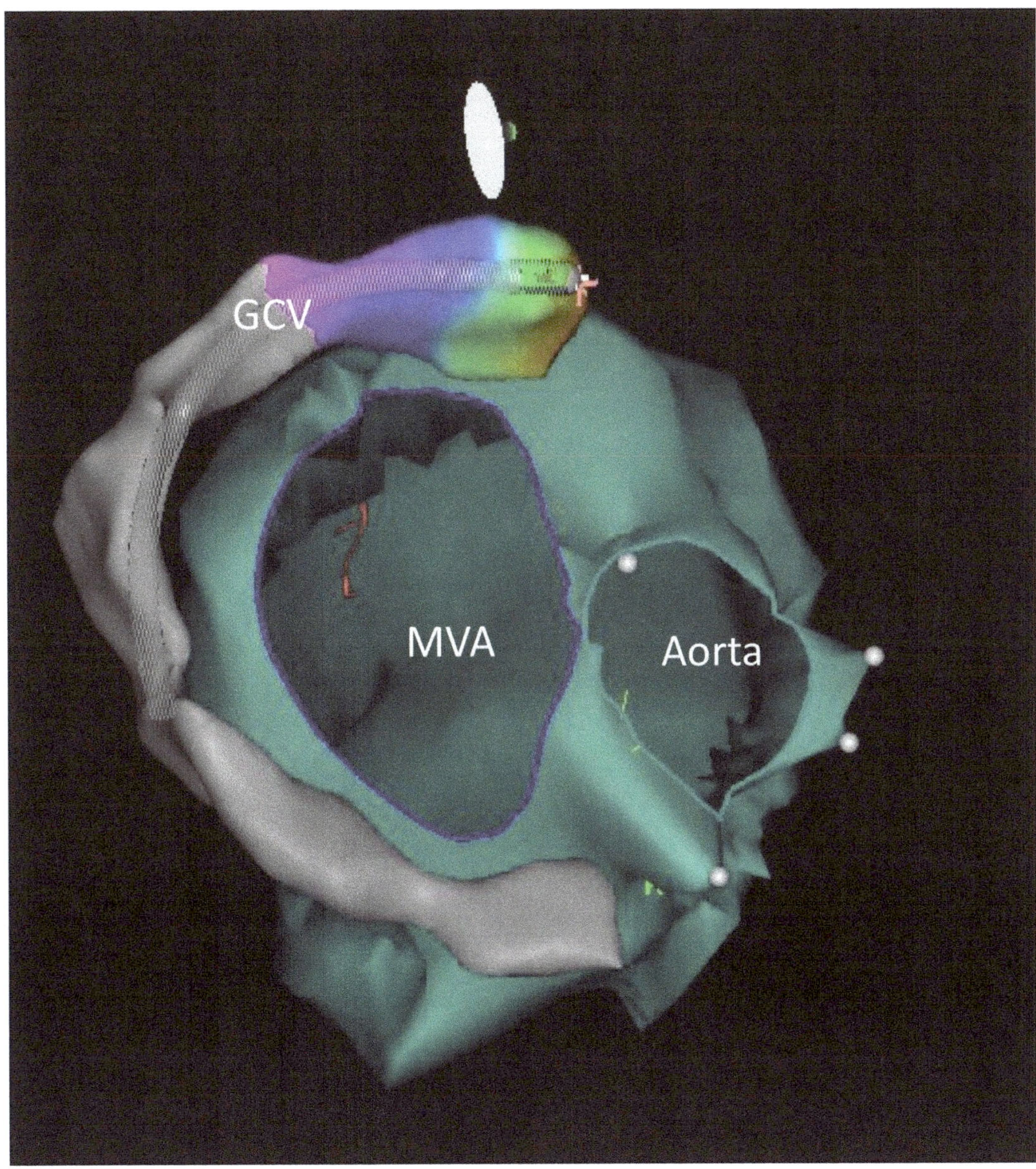

Figure 21.3 Combination of electroanatomic mapping within the GCV (EAM) and 3D echocardiographic reconstruction of the left ventricle. The GCV, the mitral valve annulus (MVA), and the aorta are labeled.

The 2D echocardiocraphic view from the intracardiac echoprobe that was placed in the RVOT is shown in **Figure 21.4**. The tip of the ablation catheter is displayed as a green icon and is located adjacent to the circumflex artery. This is too close for safely delivering RF energy.

Since this PVC was less prevalent, ablation in the great cardiac vein (GCV) was not performed.

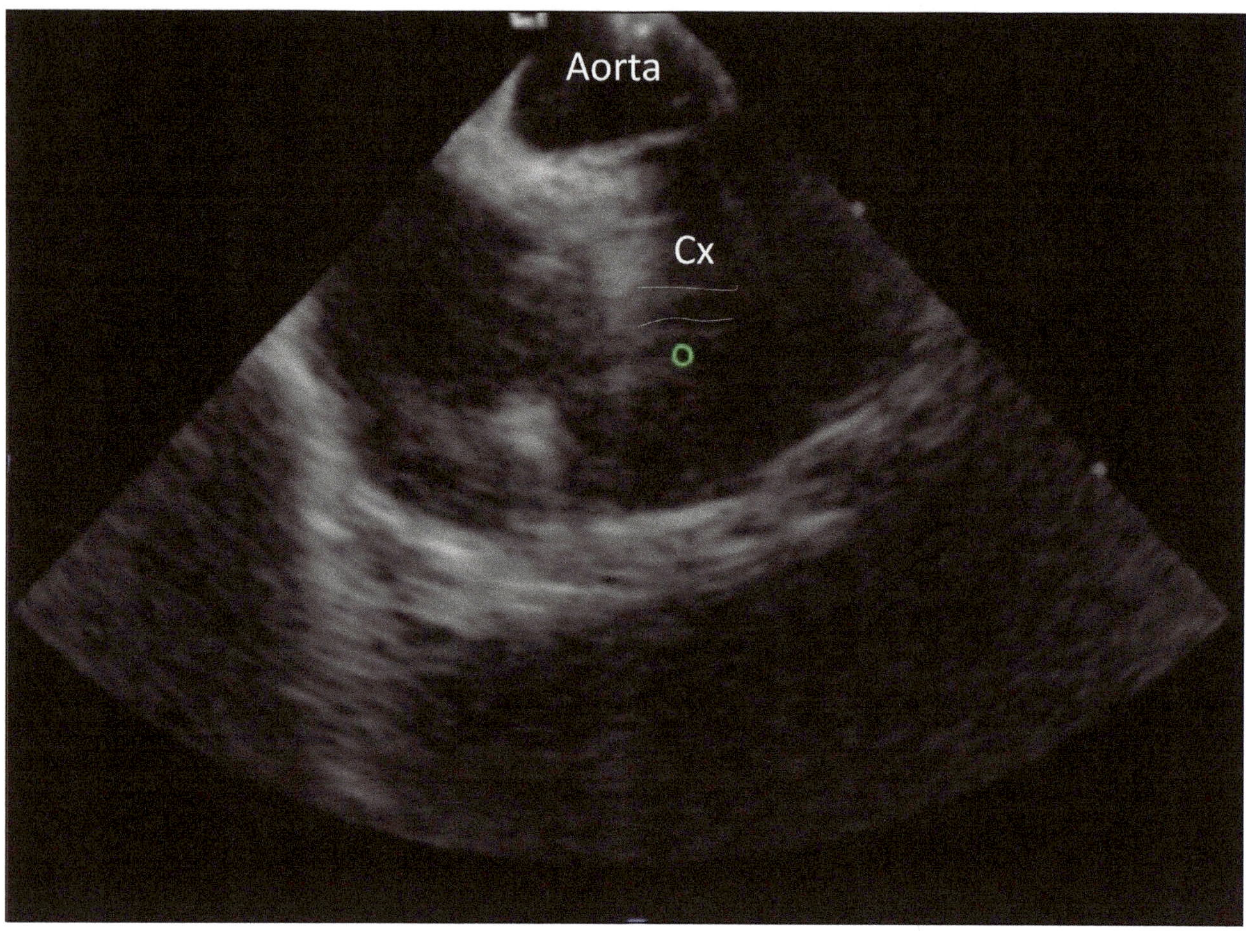

Figure 21.4 2D echocardiocraphic view from the intracardiac echoprobe that was placed in the RVOT. The tip of the ablation catheter is displayed as a **green circle**, which is adjacent to the circumflex artery, indicated with **dashed white lines**.

CLINICAL HISTORY

A 72-year-old man presented with coronary artery disease and surgical and percutaneous coronary revascularization, cerebrovascular disease with prior stroke, hypertension, dyslipidemia, and diabetes mellitus. The patient had an ICD implanted five years earlier for primary prevention of sudden cardiac death.

Over the past two months, the patient had increasing frequency of PVCs and nonsustained VT. His cardiac MRI showed midwall delayed enhancement in the interventricular septum. His ejection fraction was 15% by echocardiography.

Question

Where do the PVCs shown in **Figure 22.1** originate?

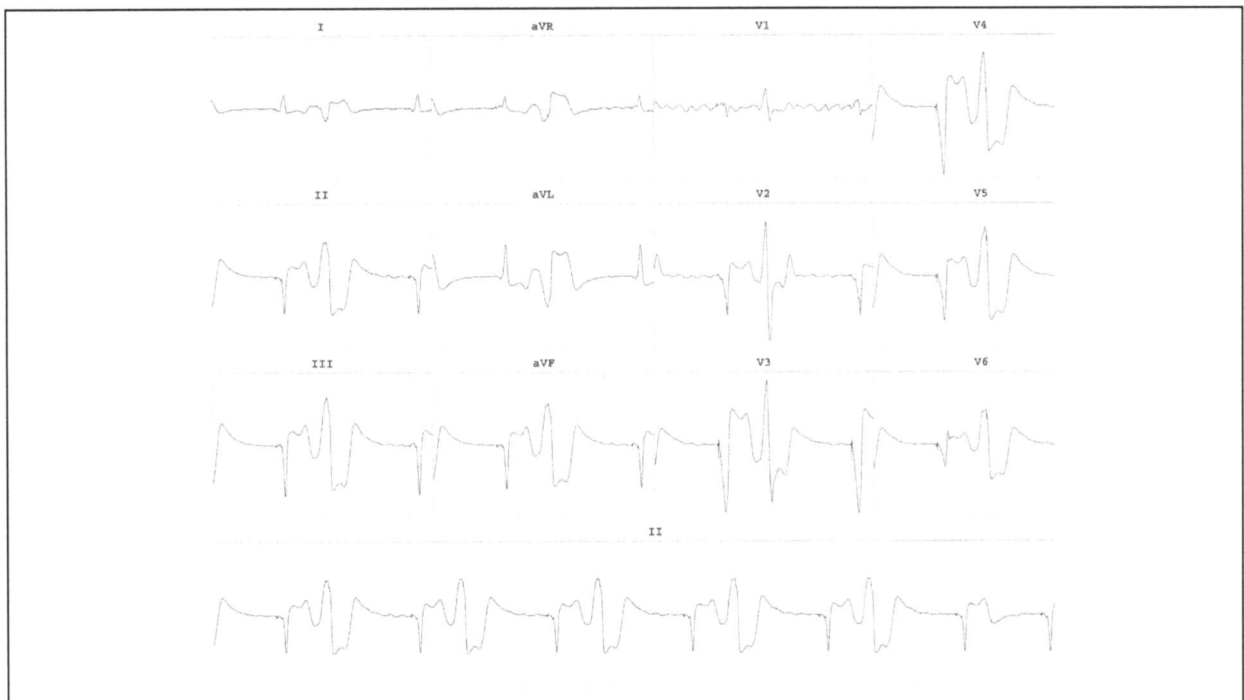

Figure 22.1   A 12-lead ECG of the patient's PVC.

Answer

The PVC originates from the commissure between the left coronary cusp (LCC) and RCC. The PVC has a W shape in lead V_1. This morphology, W in lead V_1, is often seen in cusp arrhythmias originating from the commissures. Review the following literature[1,2] and appreciate the different morphologies that are described for origins of the aortic commissures. Some of the differences may be related to electrode placements in leads V_1 and V_2.

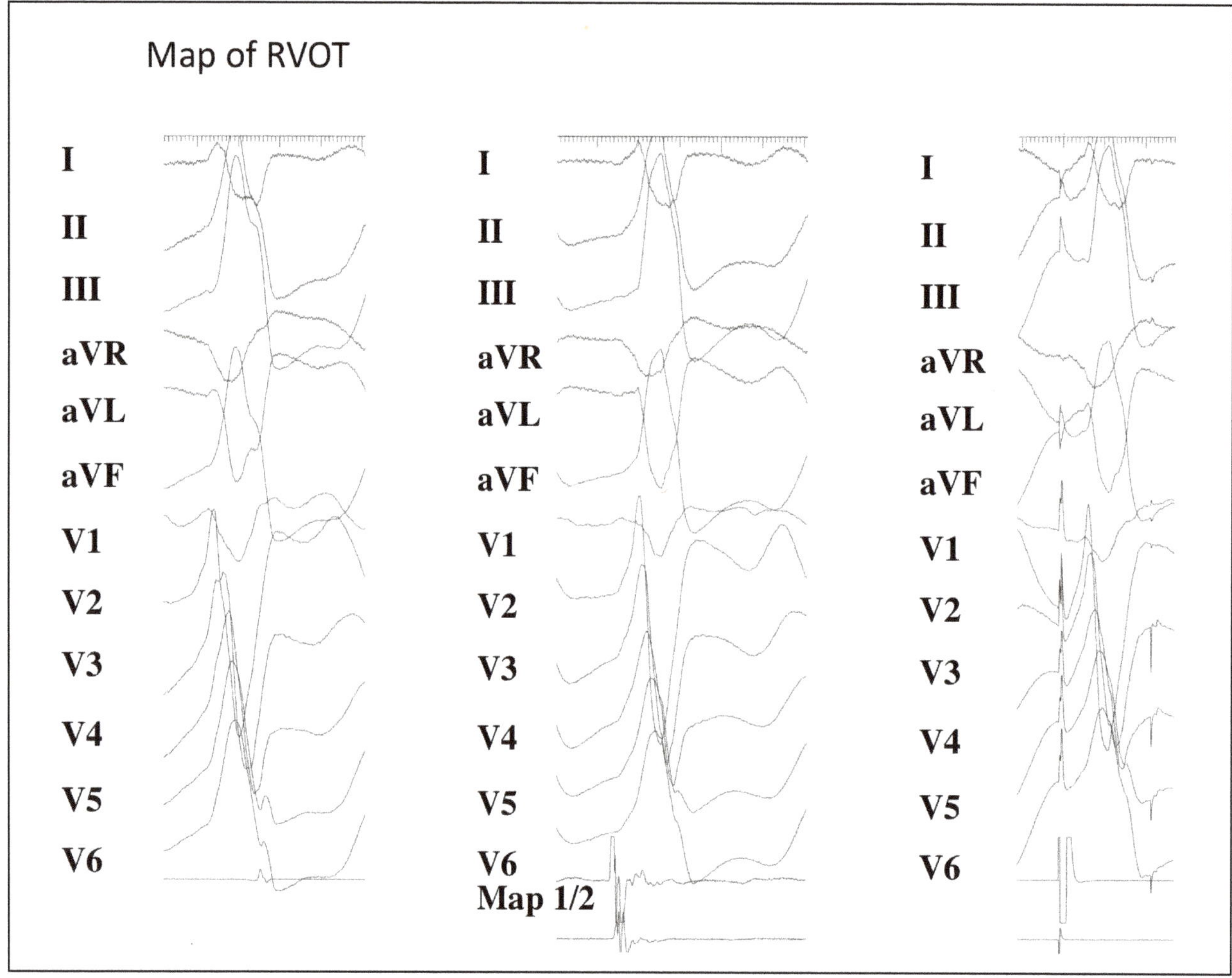

Figure 22.2 Mapping of the PVC via the RV. **Left panel:** Spontaneous PVC. **Middle panel:** The earliest activation time was −25 ms (MAP1/2). **Right panel:** Pace mapping shows a similar pace map. RF ablation from the RV was ineffective.

Ablation from the aortic aspect of the cusp failed to eliminate the PVCs and the ablation with higher power from the LV side of the commissure; angulating the catheter tip up in a J-form pattern helped to eliminate the PVC. Mapping data are shown from the RVOT (**Figure 22.2**), the aortic commissure (**Figure 22.3**), and the infravalvular area of the LVOT (**Figure 22.4** and **Figure 22.5**). Appreciate that there was no matching pace map at the successful site, indicating a deeper SOO.

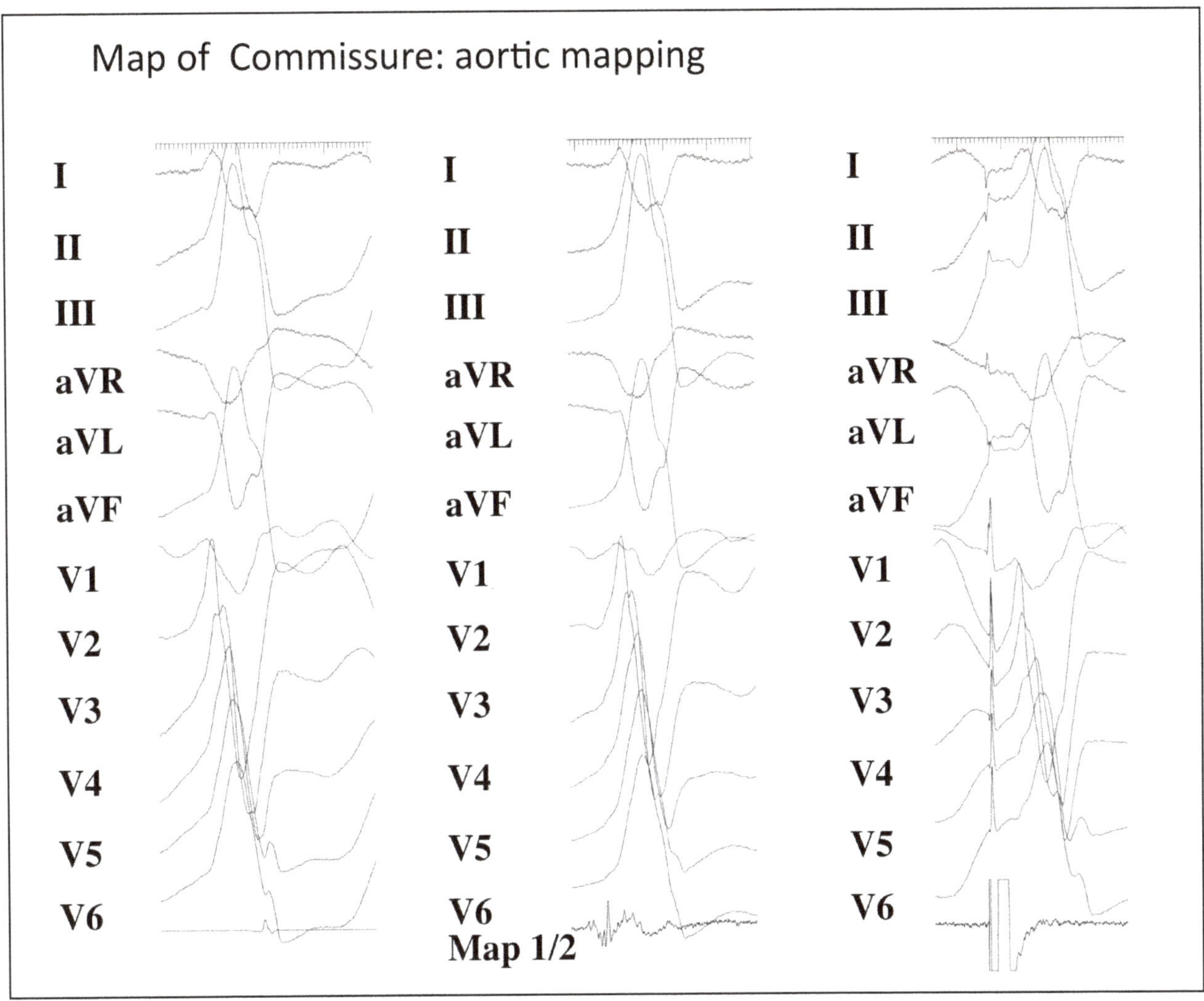

Figure 22.3 Mapping of the PVC via the aortic aspect of the commissure. **Left panel:** Spontaneous PVC. **Middle panel:** Activation time of −30 ms (MAP1/2). **Right panel:** Matching pace map. RF ablation failed to eliminate the PVC.

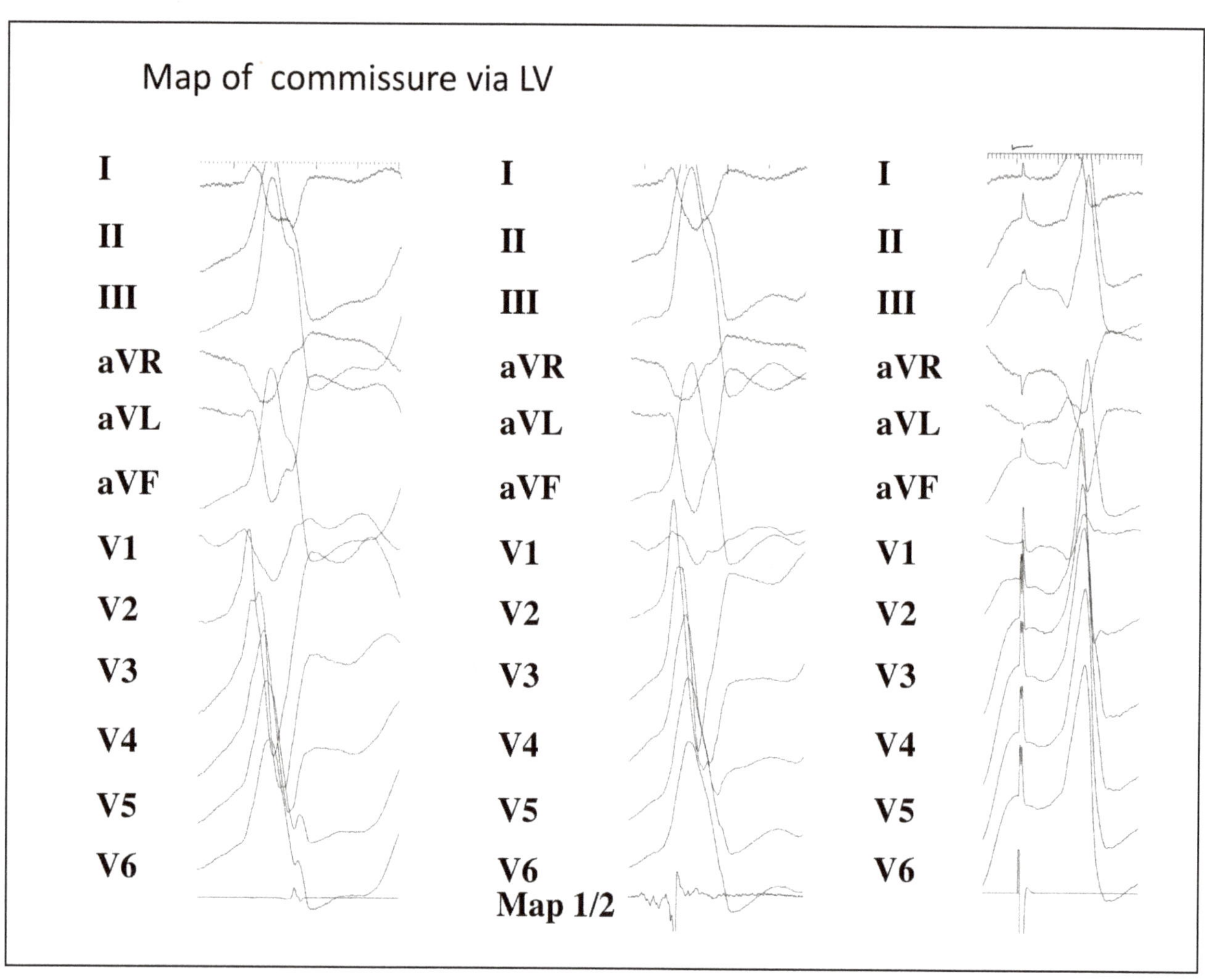

Figure 22.4 Mapping of the PVC via the LV aspect of the commissure. **Left panel:** Spontaneous PVC. **Middle panel:** Activation time of −25 ms (MAP1/2). **Right panel:** Absence of a matching pace map. RF ablation here eliminated the PVC.

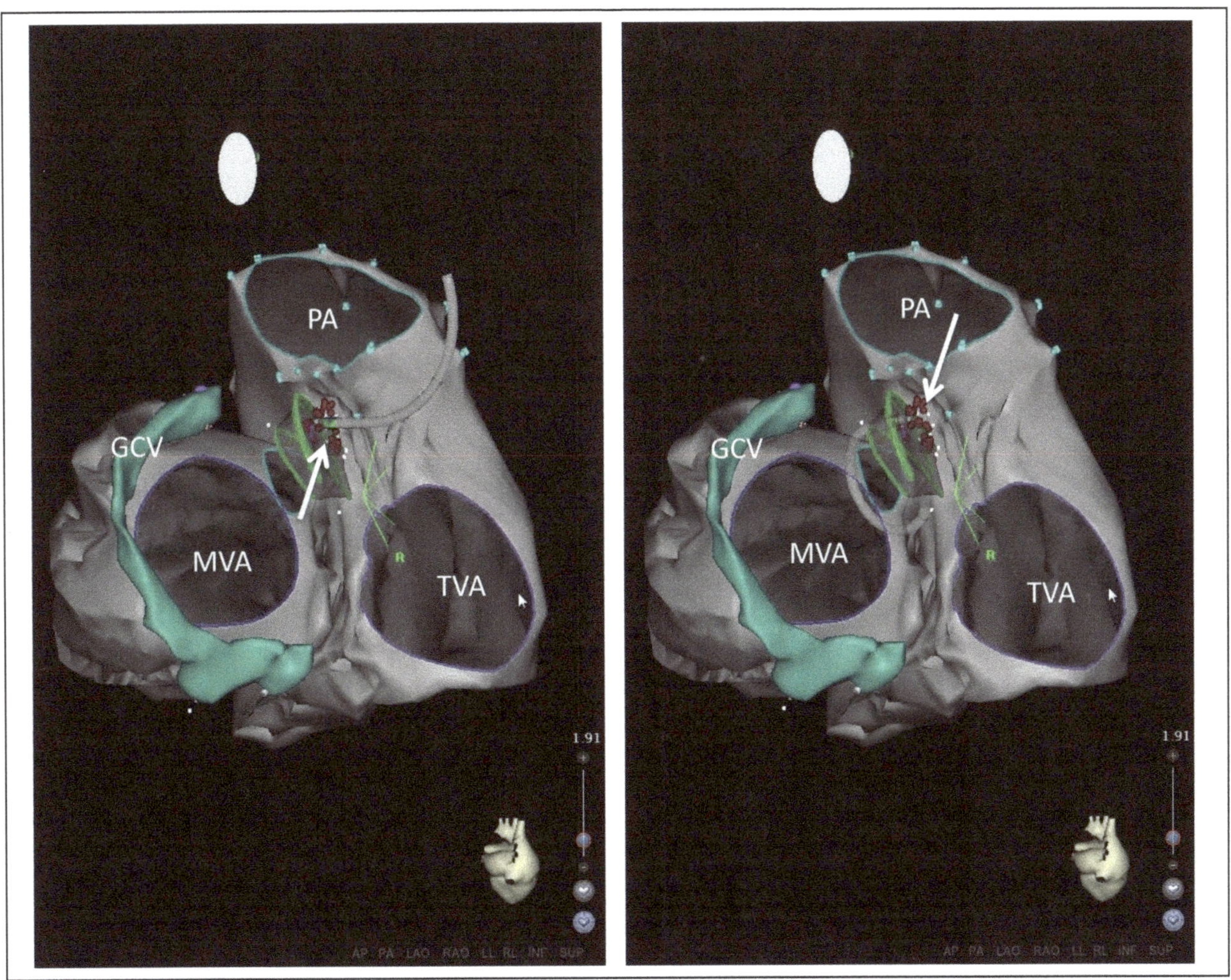

Figure 22.5 **Left panel:** 3D reconstruction of LV and RV echocardiographic contours with the catheter at the commissure accessed from the aortic aspect. **Right panel:** Same as in the left panel with the catheter accessing the commissure from the LV aspect. Pulmonary artery (PA), mitral valve annulus (MVA), great cardiac vein (GCV), and tricuspid valve annulus (TVA) are labeled.

REFERENCES

1. Yamada T, Yoshida N, Murakami Y, et al. Electrocardiographic characteristics of ventricular arrhythmias originating from the junction of the left and right coronary sinuses of valsalva in the aorta: The activation pattern as a rationale for the electrocardiographic characteristics. *Heart Rhythm.* 2008;5:184–192.
2. Bala R, Garcia FC, Hutchinson MD, et al. Electrocardiographic and electrophysiologic features of ventricular arrhythmias originating from the right/left coronary cusp commissure. *Heart Rhythm.* 2010;7:312–322.

CLINICAL HISTORY

A 63-year–old man had aortic valve replacement surgery for bicuspid aortic valve. The patient had frequent symptomatic PVCs with a PVC burden of up to 30% with normal LV function and size. He was started on amiodarone and had pulmonary side effects. The patient was referred for an ablation procedure.

Question

Figure 23.1 shows frequent PVCs in the form of couplets. Where are the PVCs originating?

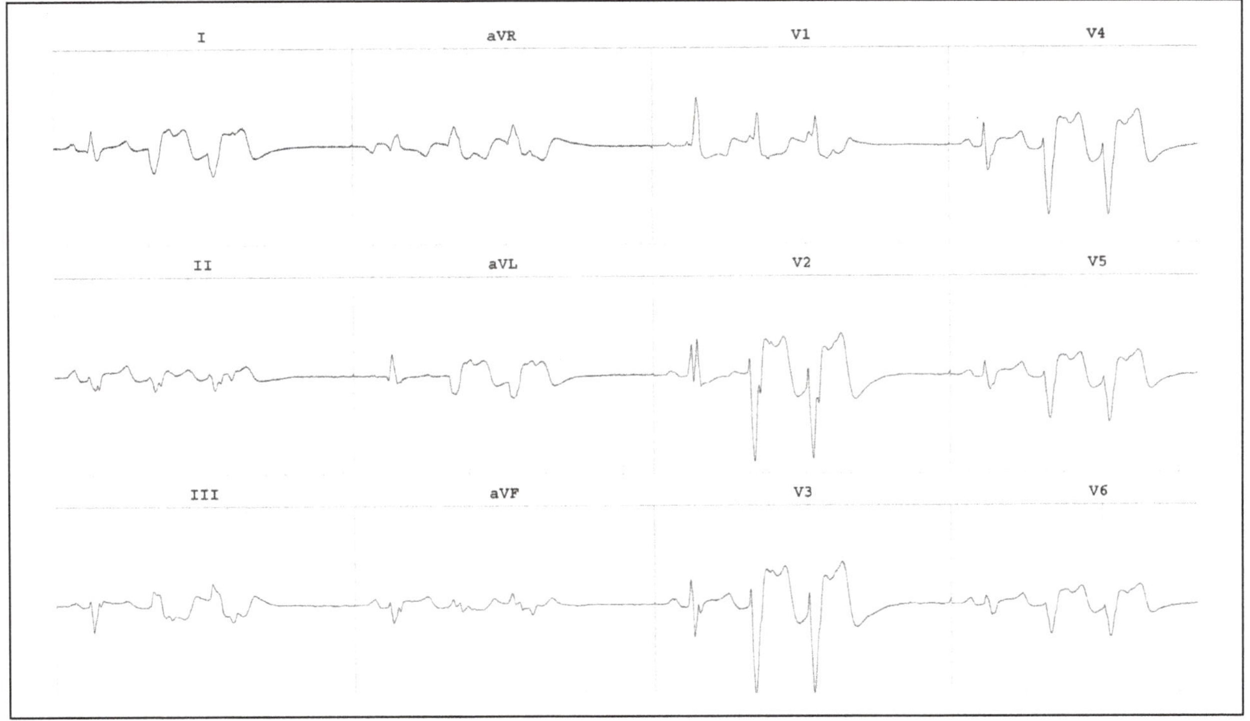

Figure 23.1 A 12-lead ECG showing a couplet.

Answer

The PVCs originate from the distal Purkinje fiber system located at the anteroapical left ventricle. A sharp potential preceded the ventricular electrogram at the SOO (**Figure 23.2**), but no Purkinje Potentials were identified during sinus rhythm beats. The SOO was localized on a trabeculation that was the extension/insertion of the posteromedial papillary

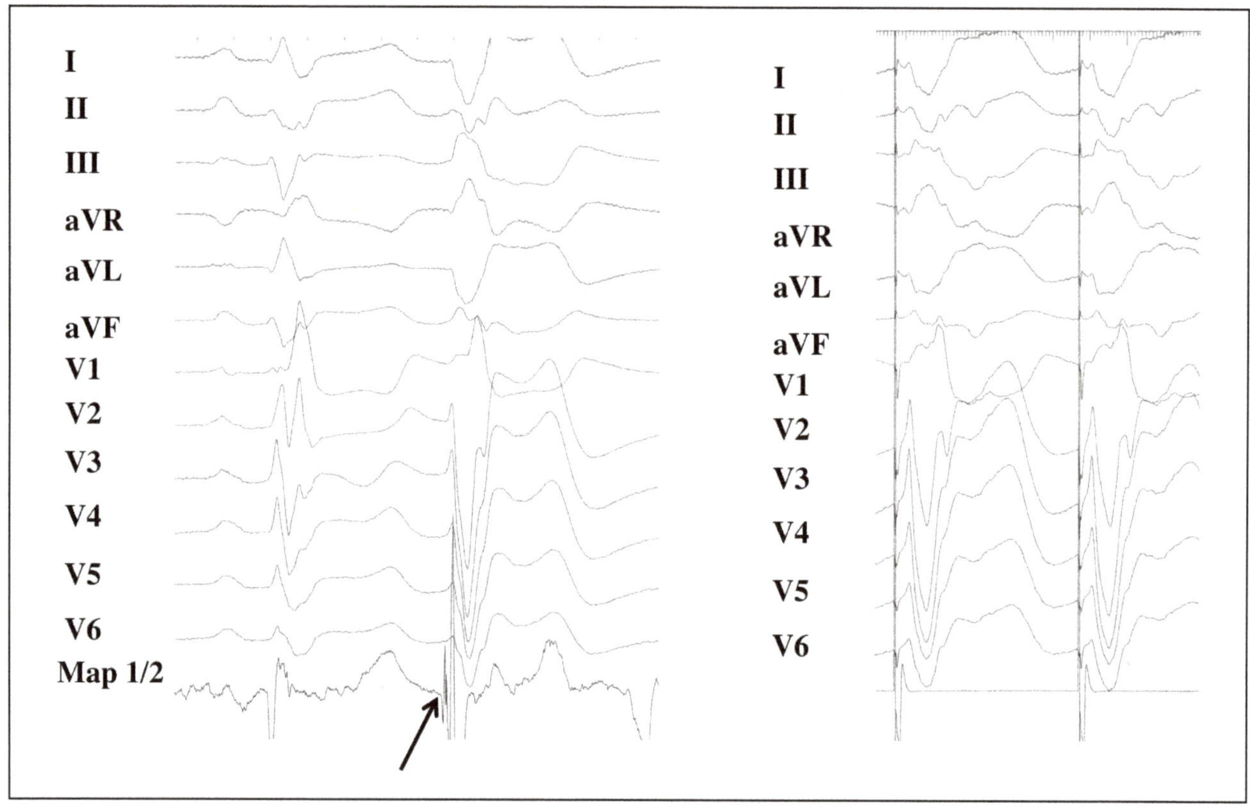

Figure 23.2   Tracings from the site of origin showing a sharp potential preceding the onset of the QRS by 20 ms (**arrow in left panel**). The pace map at this location was similar to the targeted PVC morphology (**right panel**).

muscle (**Figure 23.3**). Figure 23.2 shows a sinus rhythm QRS complex with a RBBB pattern followed by the PVC; therefore, the first QRS complex is not a PVC. The sharp initial component in V_2–V_5 supports involvement of the specialized conduction system rather than a myocardial origin.

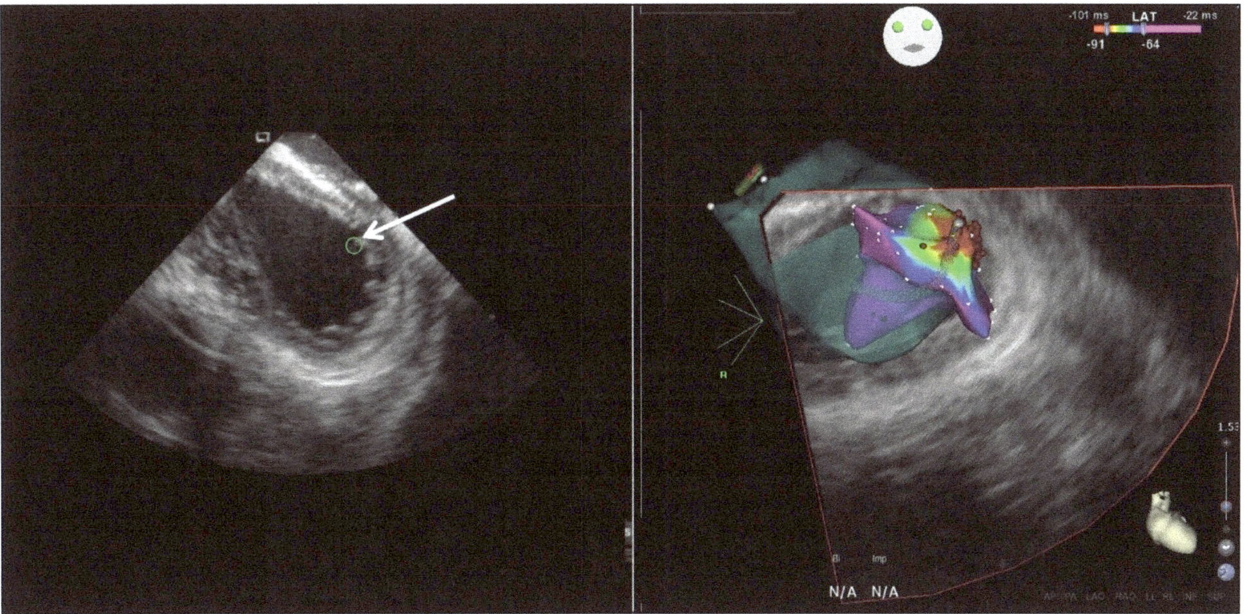

Figure 23.3 **Left panel:** Echocardiographic section through the left ventricular apex indicating the origin of the arrhythmia from one of the trabecular insertions of the posteromedial papillary muscle indicated by the locator of the catheter tip (**green circle** and **white arrow**). **Right panel:** A superimposed activation map on the echocardiography-derived shell of the left ventricular apex. The catheter position at the site of origin is shown.

CLINICAL HISTORY

A 63-year-old woman presented with nonischemic cardiomyopathy and an ejection fraction of 35%, moderate mitral regurgitation, hypertension, and prediabetes. Other than shortness of breath with mild exertion, the patient was asymptomatic. Frequent PVCs were discovered on a routine physical exam. The PVC burden was approximately 25%. A cardiac MRI showed no delayed enhancement.

Question

Where does the PVC shown in **Figure 24.1** originate from and how should the ablation be carried out?

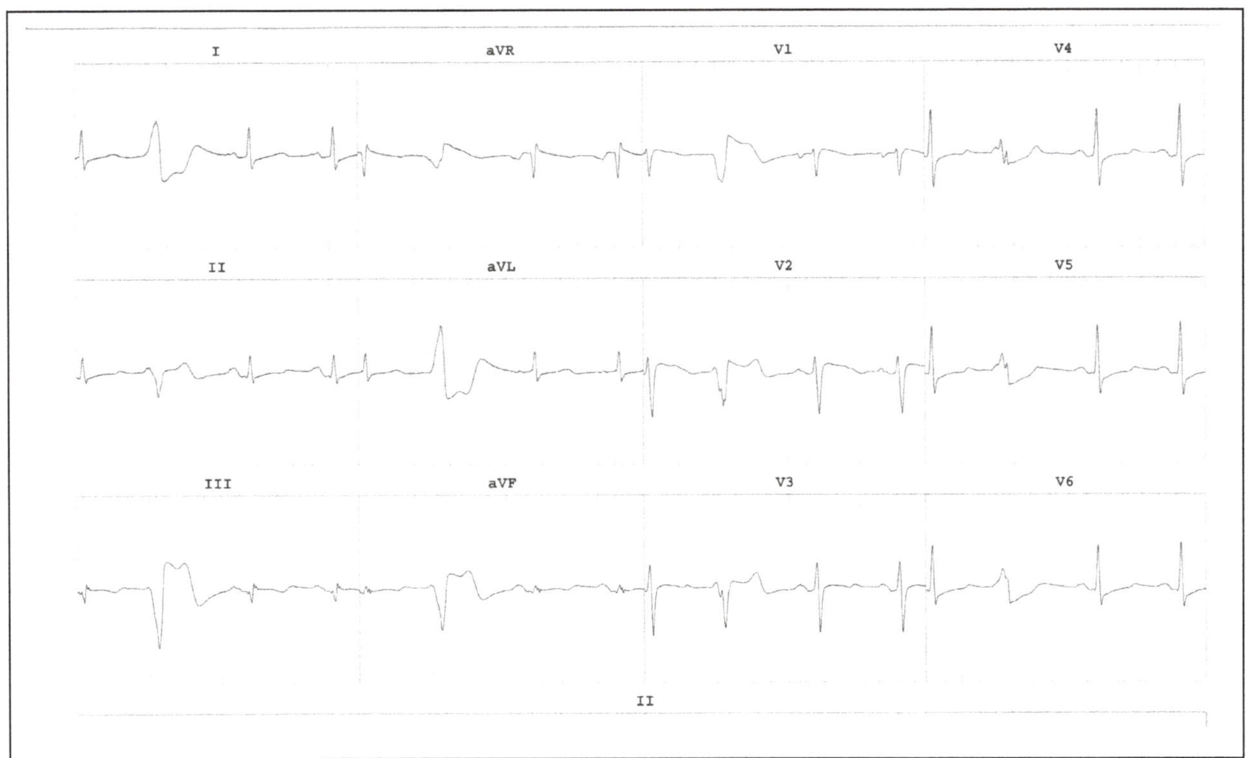

Figure 24.1 A 12-lead ECG of the patient's PVC.

The PVC originated from the parahisian area close to the slow pathway. The key features for a parahisian origin are the combination of the following: Q wave in lead V_1, tall R wave amplitude in lead I (> the inferior leads), as well as an R wave in lead aVL. In this patient, all inferior leads are negative. This often indicates that the origin is below the His bundle, and this was indeed the case. The earliest site was at a location where an atrial electrogram was also present. The atrial

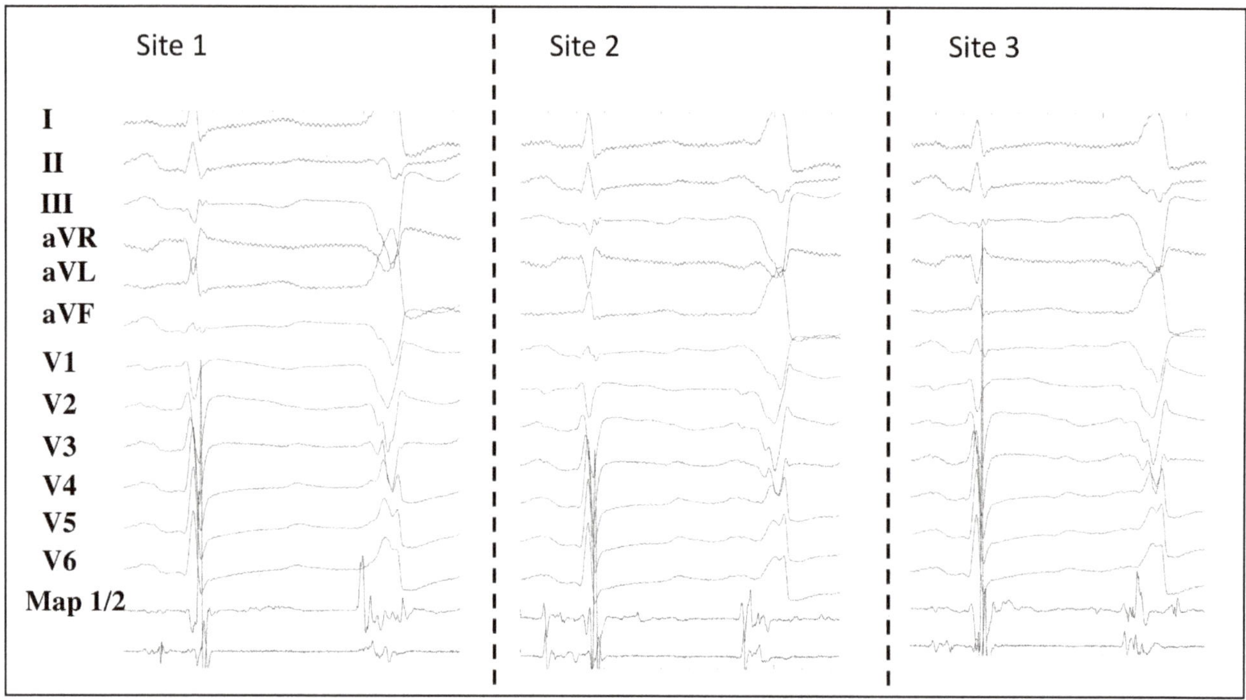

Figure 24.2 Tracings from several sites with early activation close to the His bundle. There is a small His potential at site 1 and 2 in the recordings from the distal poles (map 1/2) of the ablation catheter. At site 3, there is no His recording present, and a small atrial electrogram indicates that this is close to the slow pathway area.

electrogram was fragmented with a V:A ratio of ~4:1, typical for a slow-pathway ablation site (**Figure 24.2**). The pace map matched the PVC morphology in ≥ 11/12 leads, indicating that the SOO was close to the surface (**Figure 24.3**). During RF energy delivery below the His bundle location (**Figure 24.4**), there was a junctional rhythm typical for ablation within the slow pathway area. V-A conduction was carefully monitored during RF ablation, and PVCs were ablated without impacting on atrioventricular nodal conduction.

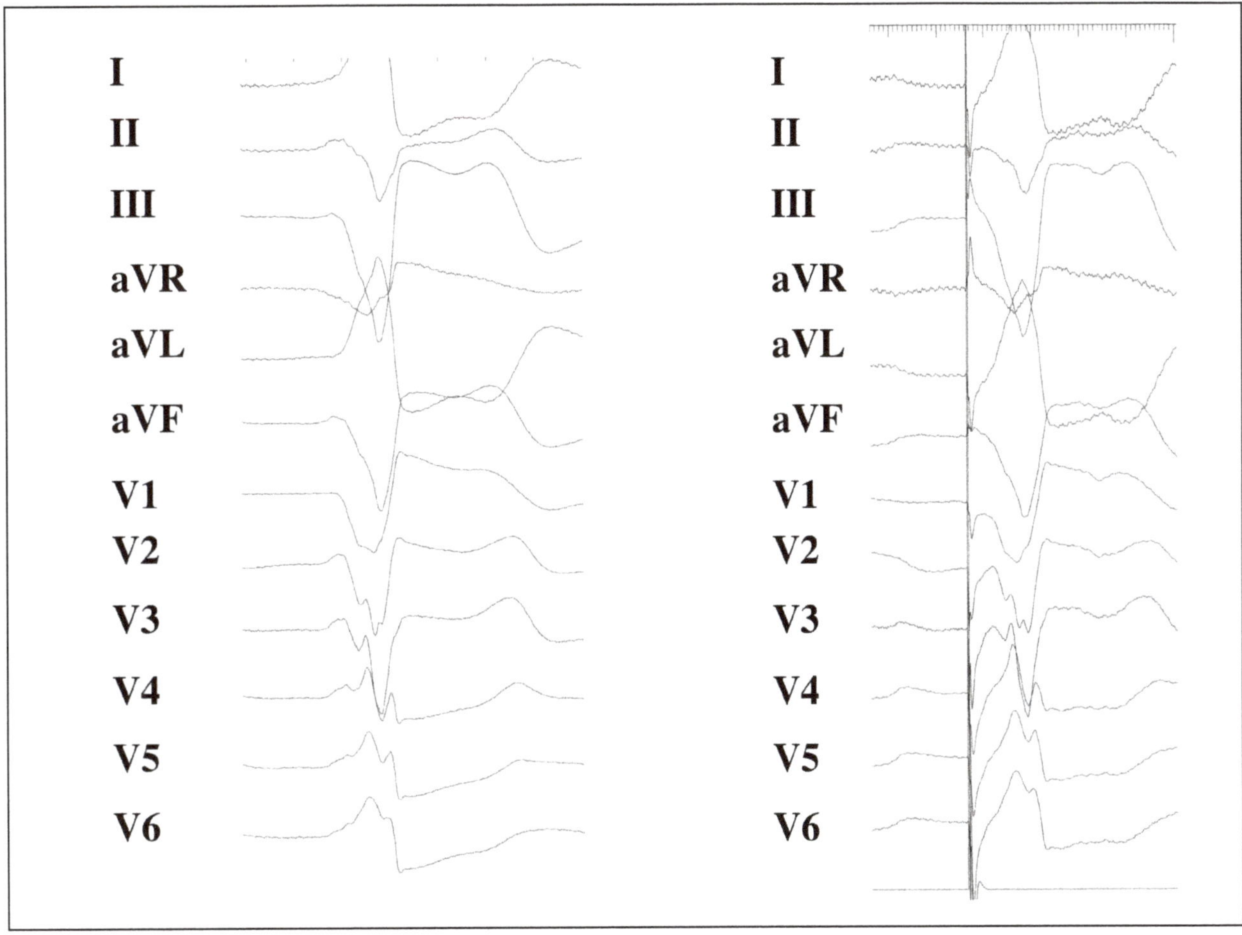

Figure 24.3 There was a matching pace map at this site (**right panel**) compared to the spontaneous PVC (**left panel**).

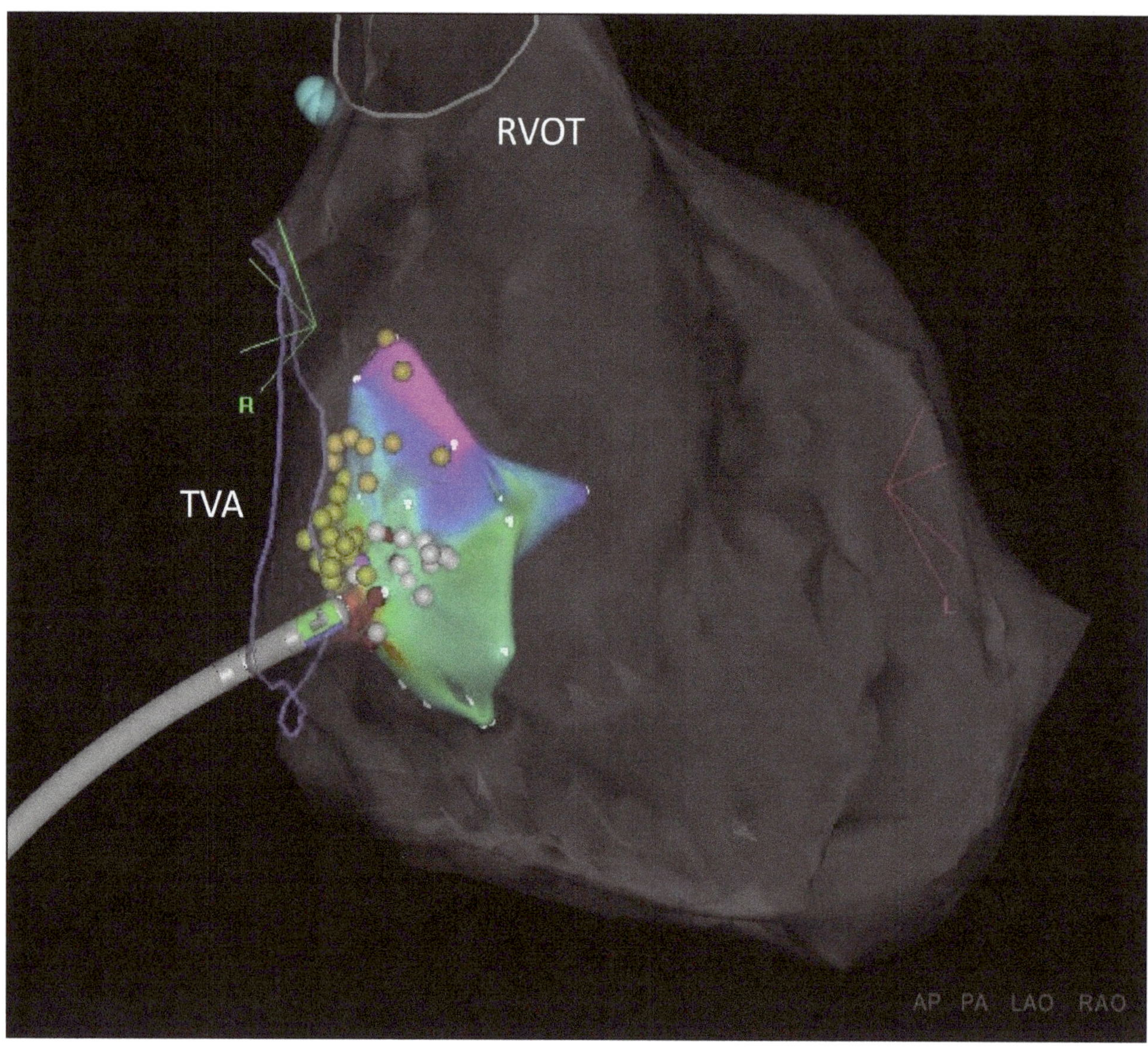

Figure 24.4 This figure shows the electroanatomic activation map fused with the 3D reconstructed shell of the right ventricle viewed from an anterior position. **Orange tags** indicate a His cloud and **red tags** indicate ablation lesions. The catheter is shown at the effective ablation site.

CLINICAL HISTORY

A 73-year-old man presented with a history of ascending aortic aneurysm and aortic root replacement sparing the aortic valve. He had frequent PVCs and had a prior PVC ablation a year earlier. His energy level improved somewhat, but his PVC burden remained elevated. A Holter showed a PVC burden of 20.5%, and on echocardiography his ejection fraction was 43%.

Question

Where do the PVCs shown in **Figure 25.1** originate, and how should they be targeted?

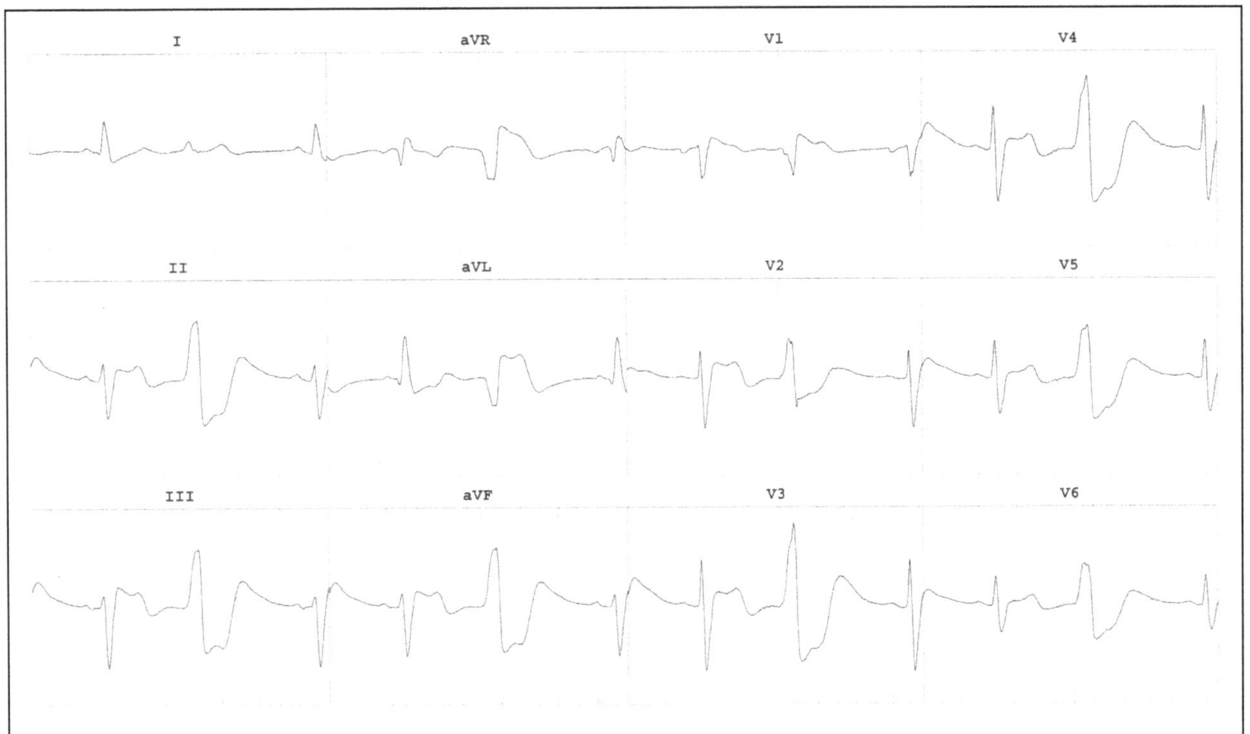

Figure 25.1   A 12-lead ECG of the patient's PVCs.

Answer

The origin was intramural. There is no obvious ECG clue to this, but during the prior procedure, RF energy was delivered intramurally via a perforator vein.

The slurred down stroke in lead V_1 might suggest an epicardial origin, but in case of an intramural origin, there may also be slower impulse propagation from an intramural origin until the propagation wavefront reaches the specialized conduction system. The predominant positive R wave in lead I argues against an epicardial origin in the LV free wall. The earliest timing was –70 ms in the first perforator vein (**Figure 25.2**). RF energy delivery at this location eliminated PVC1 and changed the morphology to PVC2, which could not be eliminated from this location, although

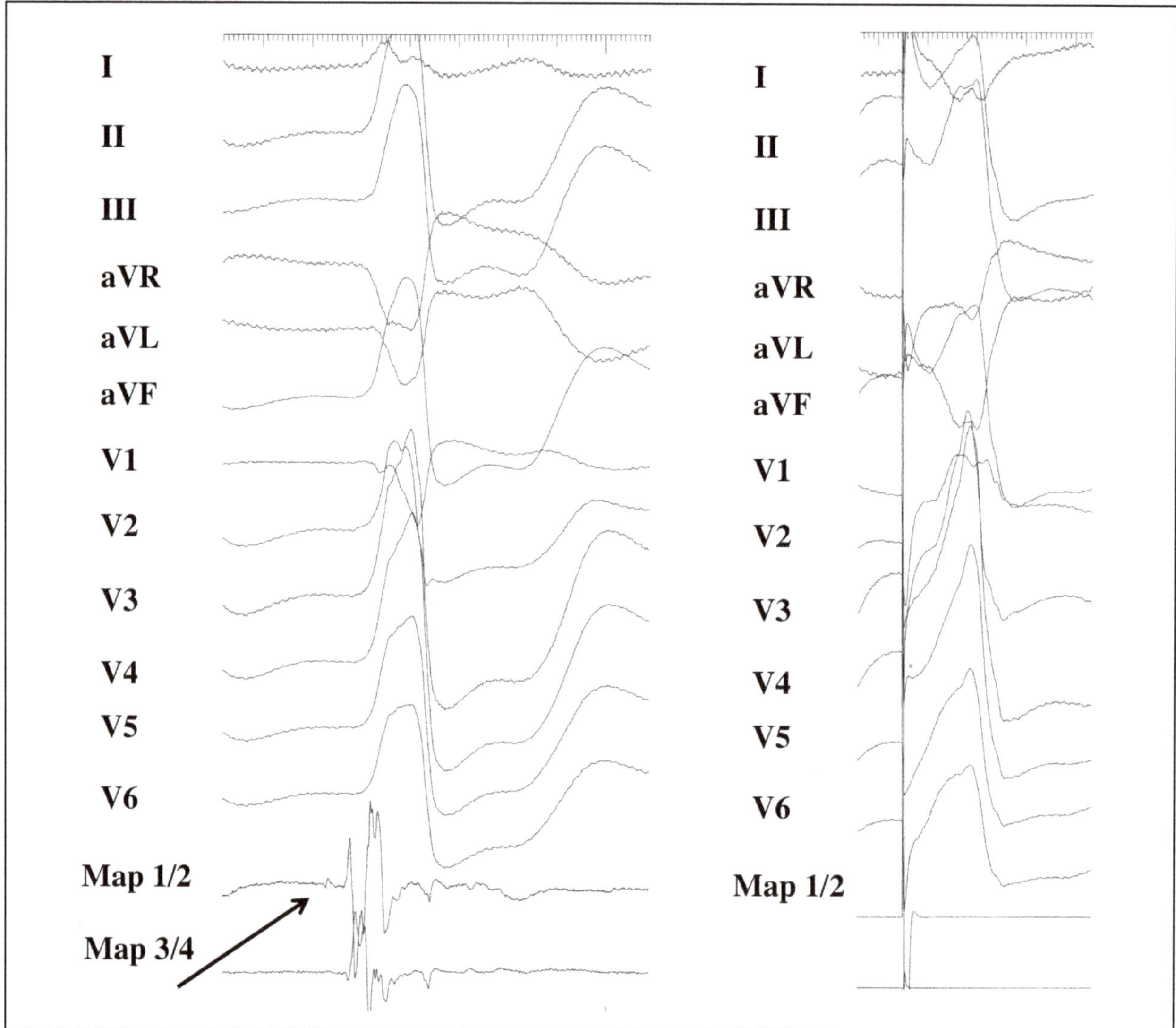

Figure 25.2   **Left panel:** Intracardiac tracings of the earliest site recorded in a septal perforator branch of the great cardiac vein. The earliest timing is –75 ms (**black arrow**). **Right panel:** Pace map at this location showed a QRS morphology that does not match with the spontaneous PVC showed in the left panel.

with pacing there was a long stimulus–QRS interval that matched with PVC2. PVC2 was mapped to the aortic cusp and the RVOT. When placing the catheter below the aortic valve and angling the catheter up towards the R/L commissure, there was early timing of −40 ms, although without a matching pace map. RF energy delivered there eliminated the PVC. In summary, this was an intramural origin with 2 different breakout sites: 1) in the epicardium close to the origin of the perforator vein (where RF energy was delivered initially); and 2) the aortic cusp, where RF energy delivery eliminated the PVC. **Figure 25.3** shows the catheter located in a perforator vein where the earliest timing was identified and where PVC1 was eliminated.

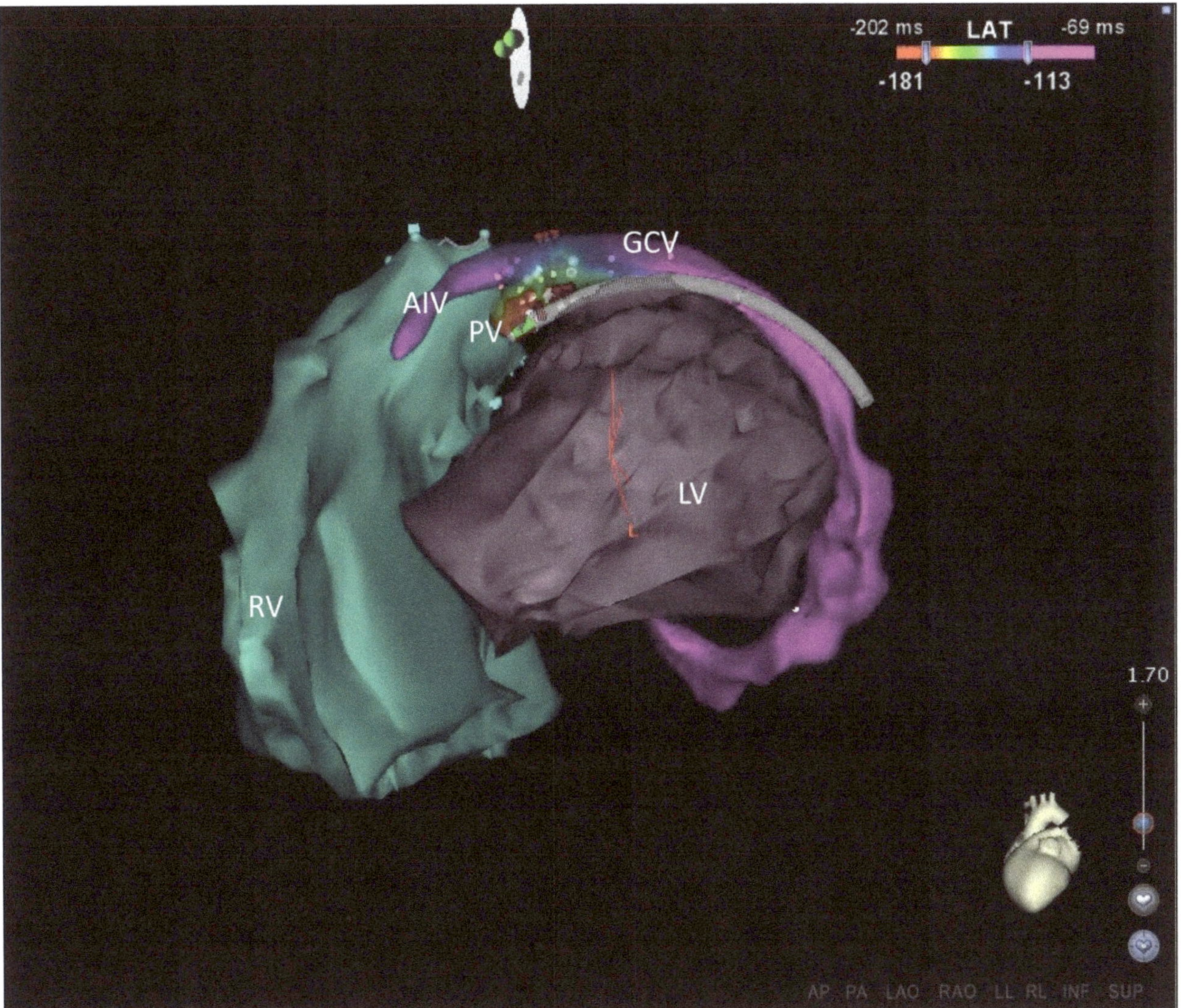

Figure 25.3 3D reconstruction of the echocardiographic endocardial shell of the left ventricle (LV) and right ventricle (RV). An activation map of the CVS is displayed on an EAM of the great cardiac vein (GCV) where the catheter was located. The anterior interventricular vein (AIV) and a perforator vein (PV) are indicated.

CLINICAL HISTORY

A 46-year-old man presented with a history of cardiac sarcoidosis, complete atrioventricular block, and sustained monomorphic VT resulting in ICD shocks. He has been on sotalol and mexiletine, but both failed to suppress his VTs. A cardiac MRI showed delayed enhancement of the septal aspect of the right ventricular outflow tract. His ejection fraction was normal.

Question

Figure 26.1 and **Figure 26.2** show two of the 10 VTs that were induced in this patient. Where do they originate?

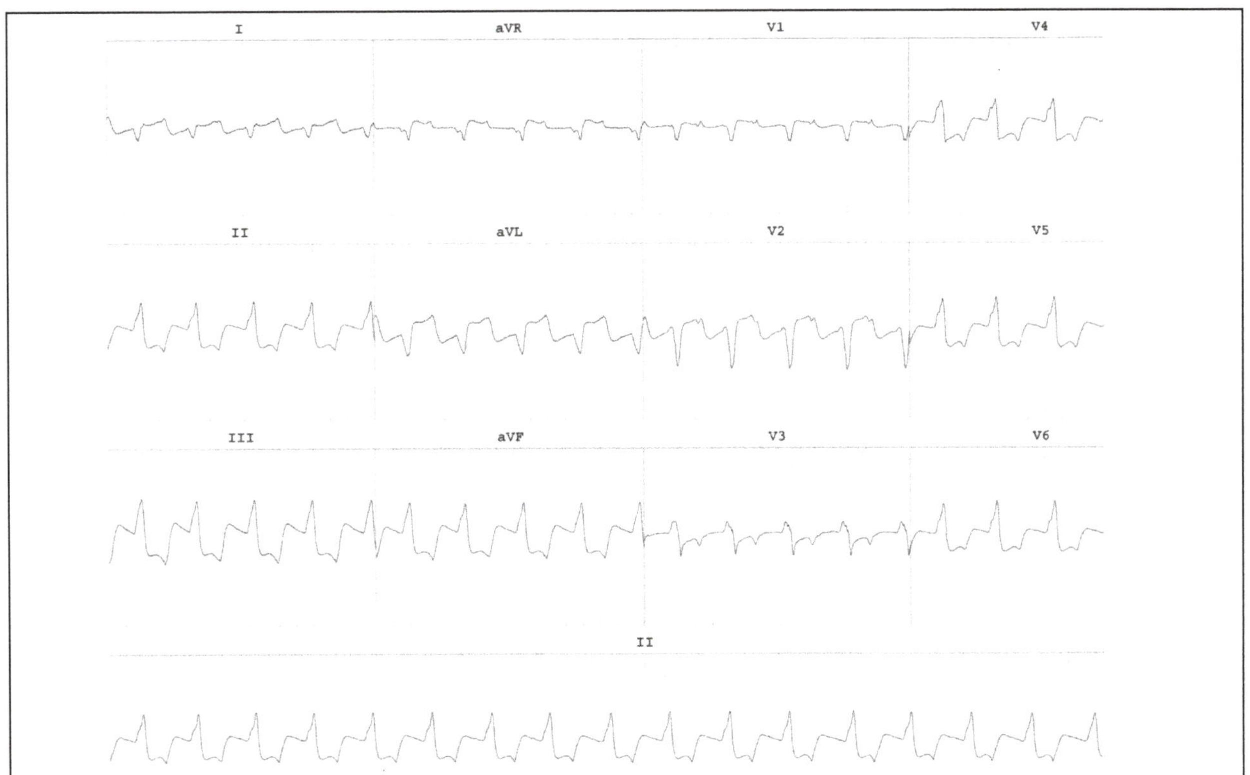

Figure 26.1　A 12-lead ECG of two induced VTs.

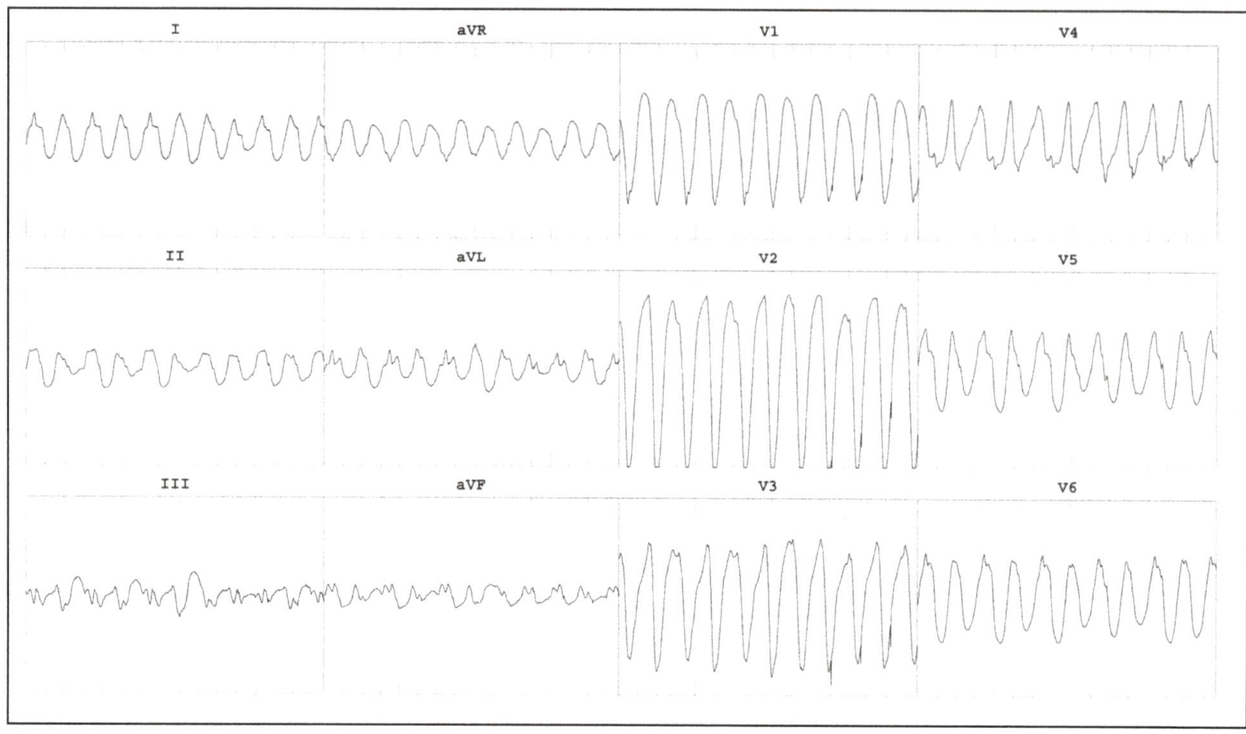

Figure 26.2 A 12-lead ECG of two induced VTs.

Answer

Both VTs originate from the septal aspect of the RVOT. The best pace maps were at a distance of 3 cm from each other. However, the morphologies are very different. Based on the 12-lead morphology, the first VT could be an idiopathic VT, a LBBBIA morphology, with a relatively narrow QRS complex. The earliest timing and the best pace map was at the anterior aspect of the septal RVOT. The second VT is much broader and has notching in the inferior leads suggestive of a free wall exit. This observation has been used to distinguish idiopathic RVOT arrhythmias from scar related VTs in patients with ARVC/D. Idiopathic RVOT VT origins more often have a narrower QRS complex because of a predominant septal origin, and VTs in the setting of ARVC/D often have a broader QRS complex due to a higher prevalence of free wall origin.[1] It is unusual to see such a discrepancy between the QRS morphologies when pacing is performed in normal tissue; this may be very different in the presence of scarring. In this patient, there was a line of block indicated by isolated potentials during sinus rhythm between the origins of both VTs. Above the line, the pace map matched for VT1; below the line, they mostly matched with the second VT. The second VT morphology suggests an origin in the basal posterior RVOT, closer to the His bundle, i.e., Q in lead V_1, tall R wave amplitude in lead I (> R wave in inferior leads and initial positive QRS in aVL. The exit sites of both VTs are shown in **Figure 26.3**.

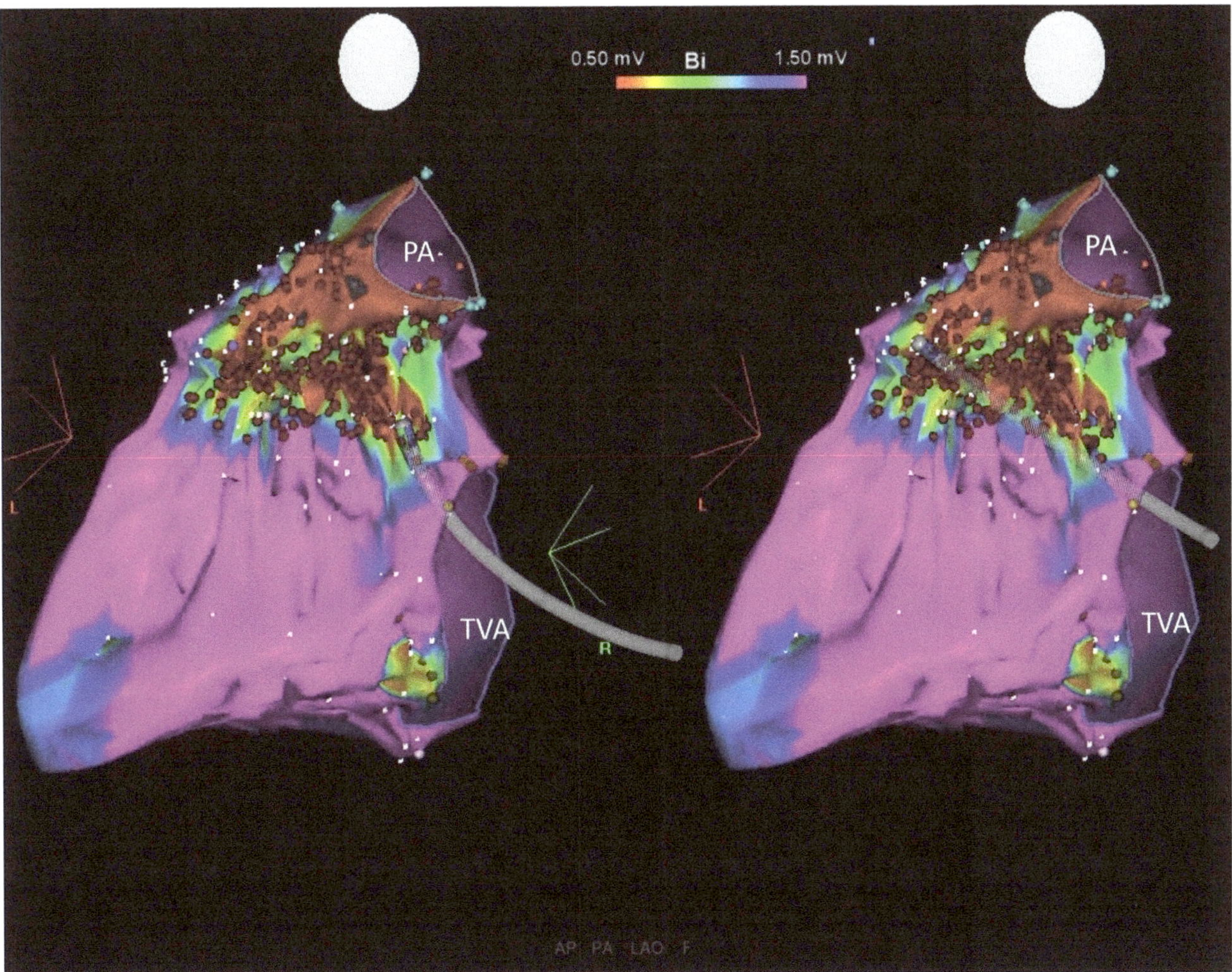

Figure 26.3 **Left panel:** Electroanatomic bipolar voltage map of the right ventricular septum with the catheter located at the site with the best pace map for VT2. **Right panel:** Electroanatomic bipolar voltage map of the right ventricular septum with the catheter located at the site with the best pace map for VT1. The sites are 3 cm apart.

REFERENCE

1. Hoffmayer KS, Machado ON, Marcus GM, et al. Electrocardiographic comparison of ventricular arrhythmias in patients with arrhythmogenic right ventricular cardiomyopathy and right ventricular outflow tract tachycardia. *J Am Coll Cardiol.* 2011;58:831–838.

CLINICAL HISTORY

A 79-year-old man with a history of symptomatic PVCs who underwent a prior ablation procedure where two PVCs were targeted. He presented for a repeat mapping/ablation procedure in the setting of ongoing symptoms, albeit with a decrease in burden from 10% to 4.5%. He had preserved biventricular function. The MRI revealed a focal area of delayed enhancement in the RV mid septum that was thought to be from the prior ablation procedure. **Figure 27.1** shows the patient's 12-lead ECG.

Question

What is the SOO of the PVC shown in Figure 27.1?

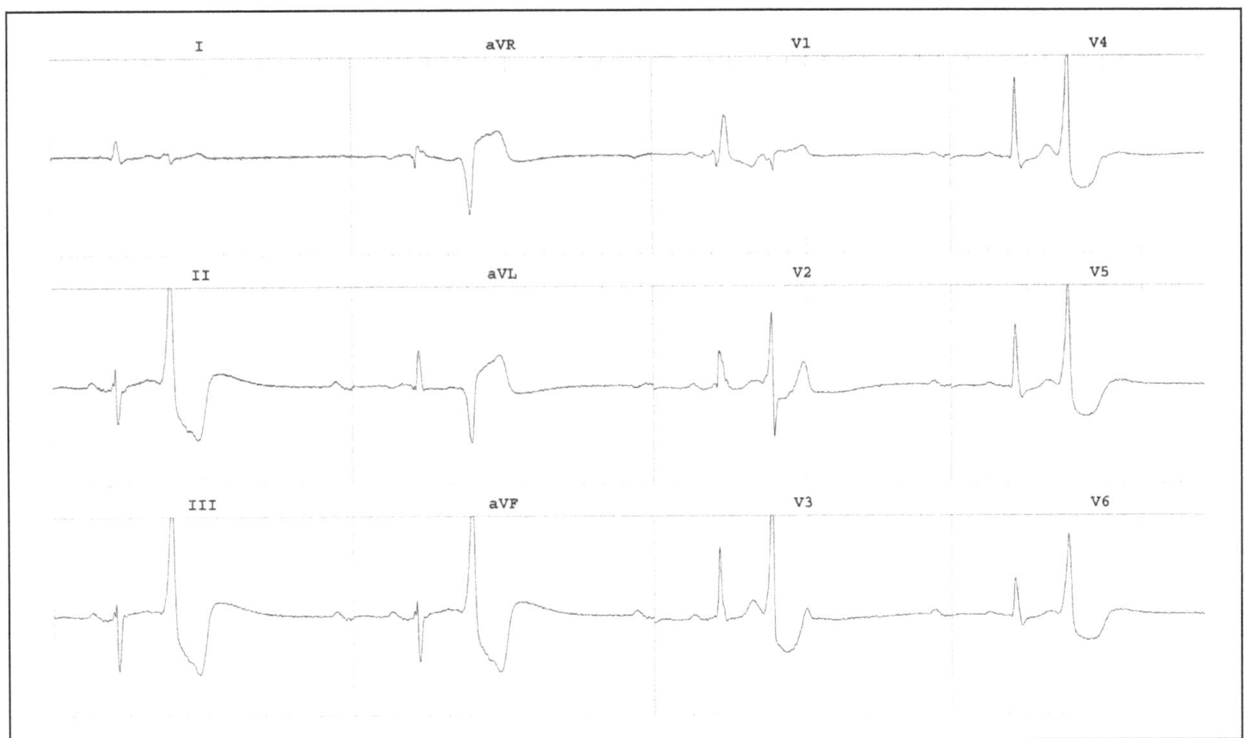

Figure 27.1 A 12-lead ECG of the patient's PVCs.

Answer

The origin was the LVOT below the aortic cusps. The morphology is somewhat unusual for the LCC. Typically, the coronary cusps are suspected if there is a LBBB morphology with an early transition ($< V_3$) and a broad R wave in leads V_1 or V_2.[1] The combination of an R wave $\geq$ 50% of the QRS and an R/S ratio $\geq$ 30% in leads V_1 or V_2 suggests an aortic cusp origin. In this case, there is no R wave in V_1 though, with a QS pattern in lead V_1. On the other hand, V_2 meets the cusp criteria. A QS pattern has been described in one series in V_1 or V_2 where the origin was the commissure between the LCC and the RCC.[2] In another series describing the same origin (commissure LCC/RCC), a Qr pattern was described,[3] casting some uncertainty on the true morphology of arrhythmias originating from the cusps and the commissures. In the series described by Bala et al., a QS pattern in V_1 was present in 15/19 patients with arrhythmias originating from the commissures and only in 2/18 ventricular arrhythmias originating from the cusps.[2]

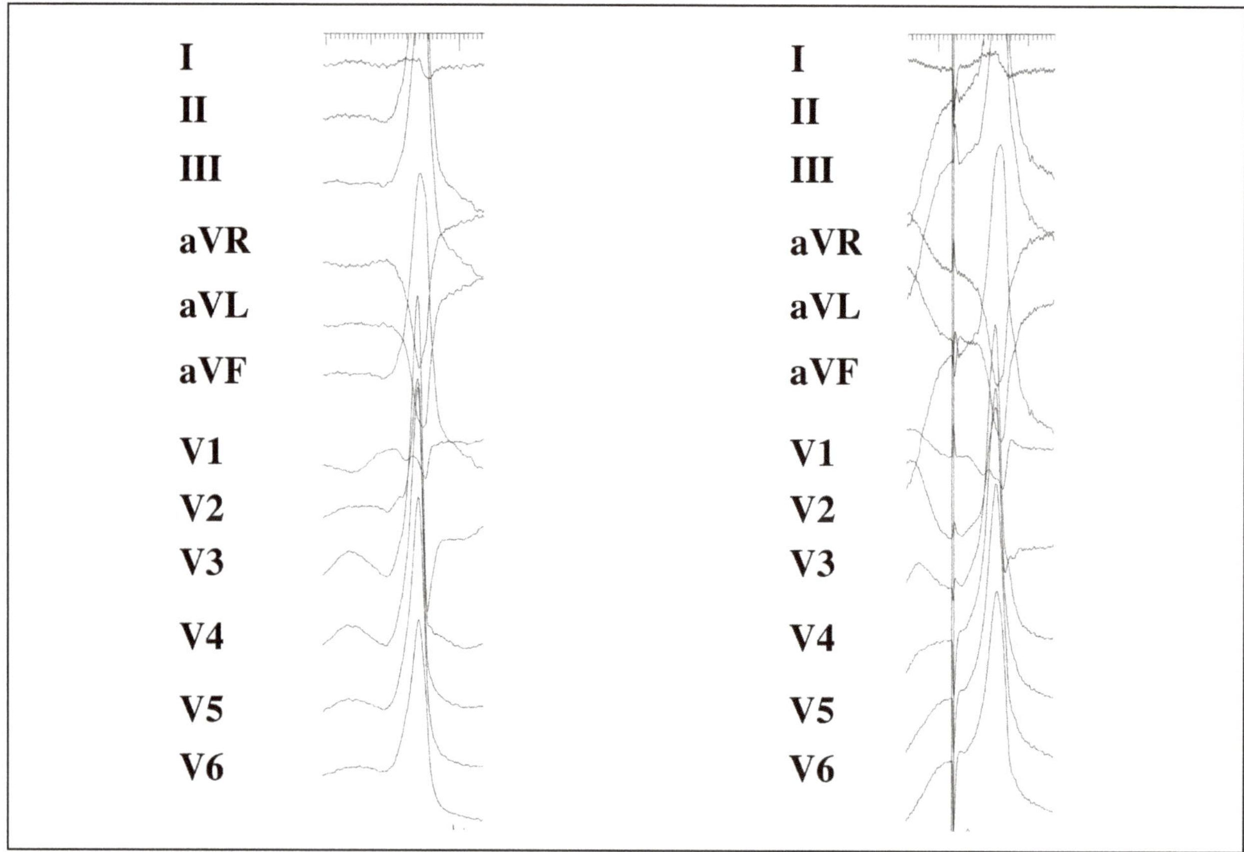

Figure 27.2 **Left panel:** Intracardiac tracings from the left coronary cusp (aortic surface). **Right panel:** Pace map showing a matching pace map for the spontaneous PVC.

In this patient, we were surprised that we had closely but not perfectly matching pace maps in the LCC (**Figure 27.2**). An ablation was attempted in the LCC during a prior procedure, and therefore the local electrograms had a farfield appearance (**Figure 27.3**). Ablation there failed to eliminate the PVCs. We then placed the catheter below the aortic cusp deflecting the tip up with a J-shaped curve. The electrograms had a farfield character and the proximal electrodes showed earlier activation than the distal electrodes (Figure 27.3). By relaxing the J curve a little bit, the catheter reached a more proximal position in the LVOT with the earliest timing, and RF energy delivery there eliminated the PVCs (**Figure 27.4**). Therefore, the origin was in proximity of the LCC/LVOT. In a prior report, supravalvular LVOT arrhythmias were compared to infravalvular LVOT arrhythmias, and the presence of an S wave in V_5/V_6 favored an infraaortic origin.[4] However, this is not the case here. Ouyang et al. suggested that ventricular outflow tract arrhythmias originating from the LVOT below the aortic cusps are characterized by a Q-wave amplitude in aVL > aVR and a III / II R-wave ratio > 1.1.[5] This was the case here as well.

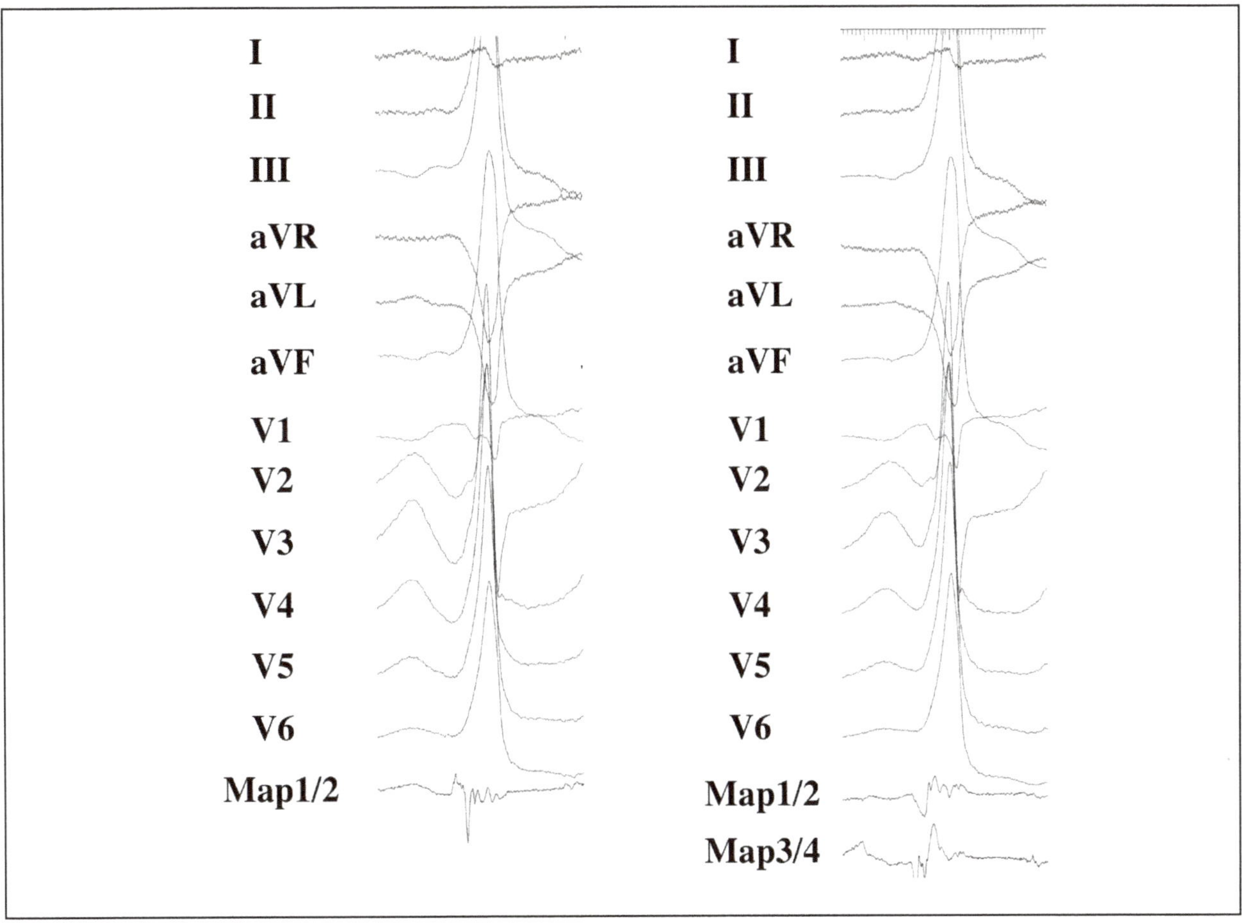

Figure 27.3 **Left panel:** Recordings from the LCC. **Right panel:** Recordings from the LVOT.

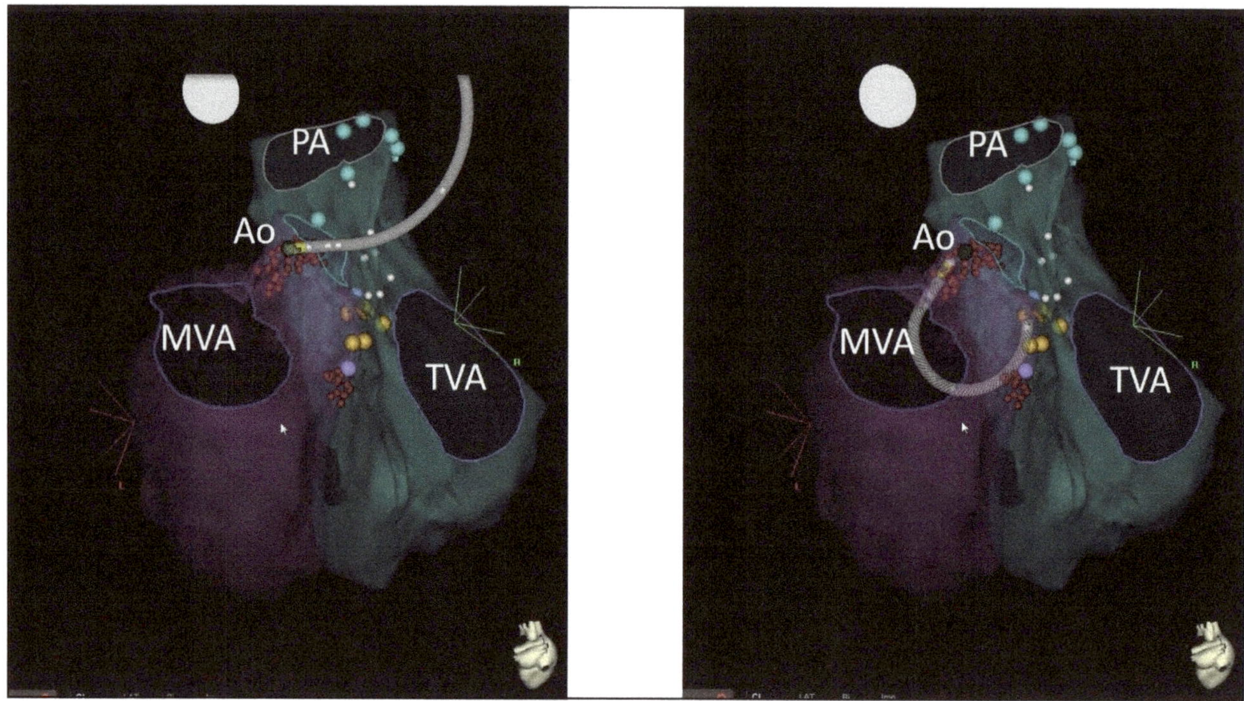

Figure 27.4 3D reconstruction of echocardiographic shells of the right and left ventricles (RV and LV) fused with mapping points of the electroanatomic map. **Left panel:** Cather positioned in the left cusp. The mitral valve annulus (MVA), tricuspid valve annulus (TVA), aortic valve (Ao), and the pulmonary artery (PA) are labeled.

REFERENCES

1. Ouyang F, Fotuhi P, Ho SY, et al. Repetitive monomorphic ventricular tachycardia originating from the aortic sinus cusp: Electrocardiographic characterization for guiding catheter ablation. *J Am Coll Cardiol.* 2002;39:500–508.
2. Bala R, Garcia FC, Hutchinson MD, et al. Electrocardiographic and electrophysiologic features of ventricular arrhythmias originating from the right/left coronary cusp commissure. *Heart Rhythm.* 2010;7:312–322.
3. Yamada T, Yoshida N, Murakami Y, et al. Electrocardiographic characteristics of ventricular arrhythmias originating from the junction of the left and right coronary sinuses of valsalva in the aorta: The activation pattern as a rationale for the electrocardiographic characteristics. *Heart Rhythm.* 2008;5:184–192.
4. Hachiya H, Aonuma K, Yamauchi Y, et al. Electrocardiographic characteristics of left ventricular outflow tract tachycardia. *Pacing Clin Electrophysiol.* 2000;23:1930–1934.
5. Ouyang F, Mathew S, Wu S, et al. Ventricular arrhythmias arising from the left ventricular outflow tract below the aortic sinus cusps: Mapping and catheter ablation via transseptal approach and electrocardiographic characteristics. *Circ Arrhythm Electrophysiol.* 2014;7:445–455.

CLINICAL HISTORY

A 68-year-old man presented with VT in the setting of ischemic cardiomyopathy (chronically occluded left anterior descending artery), congestive heart failure, renal dysfunction, sleep apnea, and chronic obstructive pulmonary disease (COPD). His arrhythmia history was significant because of persistent atrial fibrillation and recurring VT with appropriate ICD (CRT-D system) therapies. His MRI revealed extensive scarring involving the anterior and apical regions. His ejection fraction was depressed at 15%.

Question

A 12-lead ECG (**Figure 28.1**) shows one of his inducible VTs. Where does it originate?

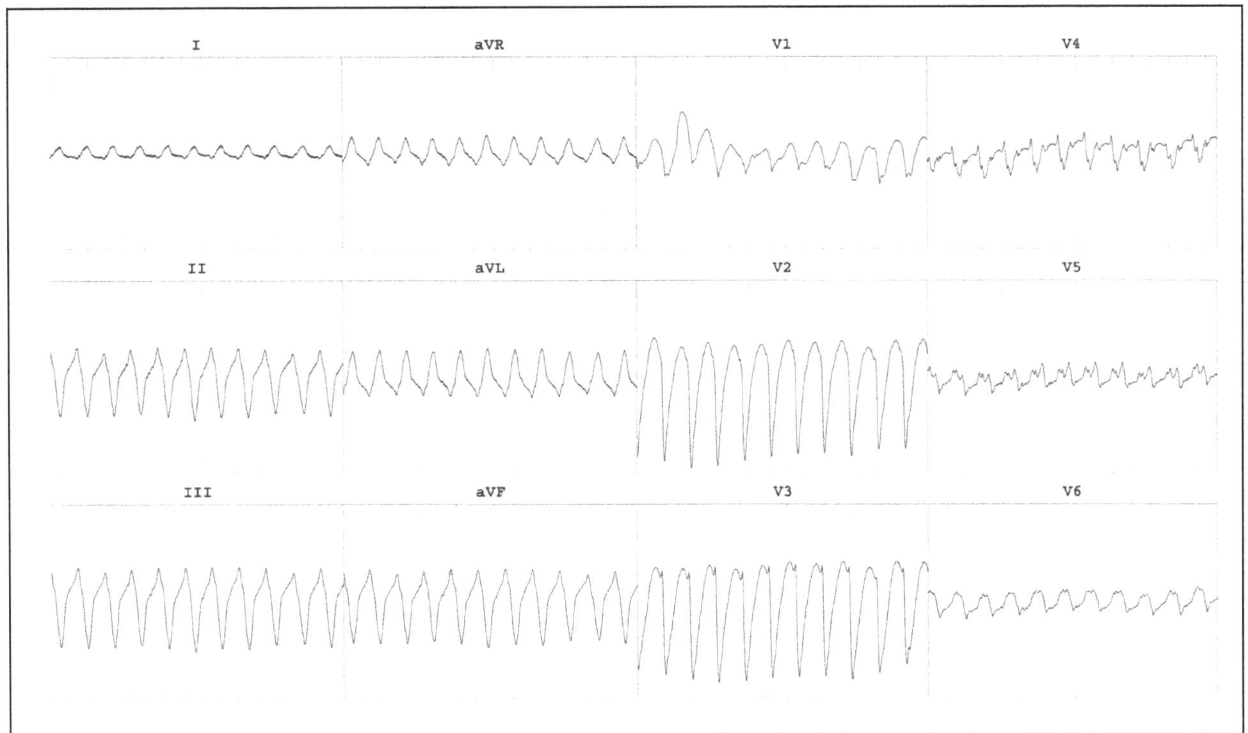

Figure 28.1 A 12-lead ECG of the patient's VT.

Answer

The origin of the VT was the scar located in the high interventricular septum. In postinfarction patients, a LBBB VT most often originates in the interventricular septum. Typically, scarring involves the septum and often the VTs are successfully ablated from the LV, especially if mapping can be performed during tachycardia. If the VT is not tolerated, as in the case of this patient, the exit site can be identified by pace mapping. The best pace maps were found in the RV septum. The initial QRS axis is inferiorly directed, although this is difficult to appreciate with the rapid rate, and all of the initial QRS complexes in the inferior leads are positive (although there is an S wave present at the end of the QRS complex merging with the T wave, see **Figure 28.2**). One would not necessarily expect this VT to originate from the septum, because the QRS complex is very broad. However, the LV in this patient is not normally activated transseptally, and activation of the LV occurs later, most likely due to the presence of extensive septal scarring. This may

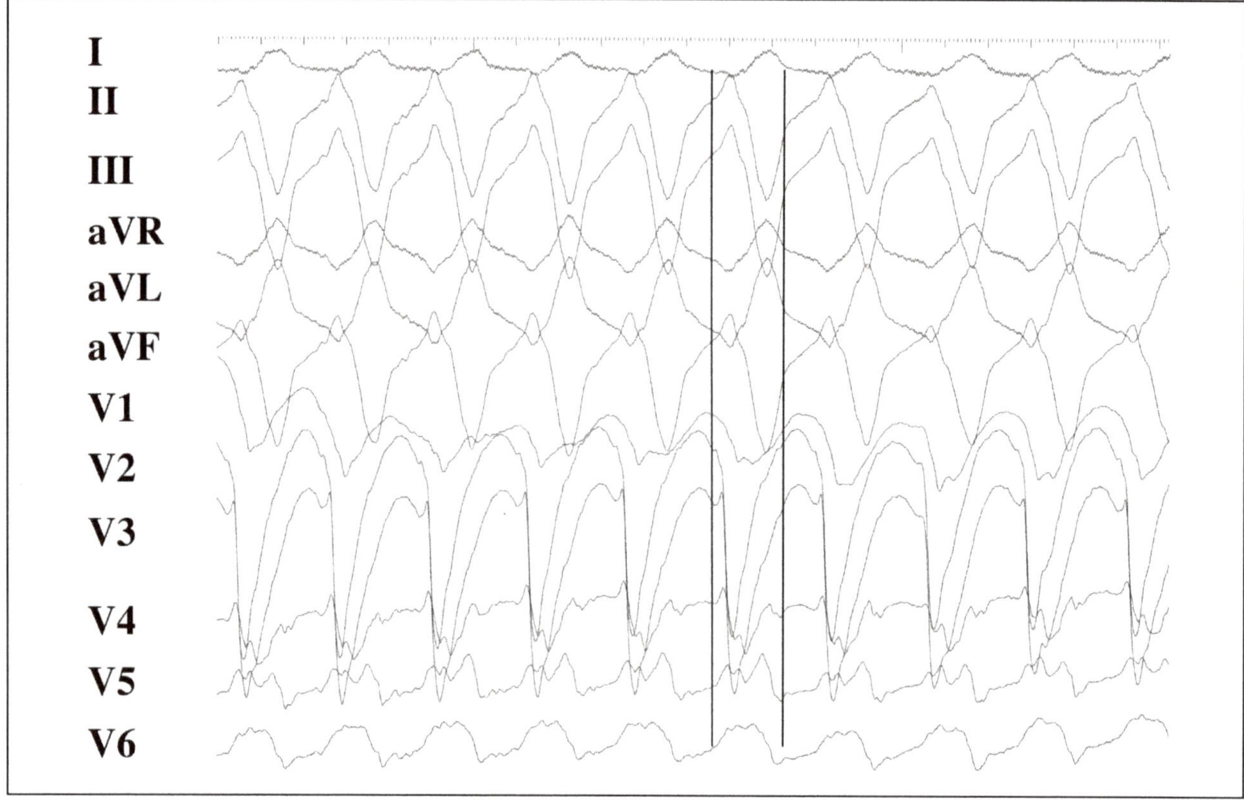

Figure 28.2 A 12-lead ECG displaying all 12-lead ECG tracings at the same time. The two vertical lines indicate the beginning and the end of a VT-QRS complex.

explain the late transition. A late transition in these post-myocardial infarction (MI) VTs does not distinguish LBBB VTs that have a RV exit from VTs with a LV exit. A prior manuscript failed to identify ECG characteristics that favored a RV as opposed to a LV septal exit.[1] In postinfarction patients in whom the RV septum is part of the VT circuit, the EF is lower, and they often have had a prior anterior wall infarction compared to patients with septal involvement in whom there is no RV involvement.[1] In more than half of the patients with septal infarction, the right ventricular septum harbors critical areas of inducible postinfarction VTs.[1] In postinfarction patients where critical RV sites were identified, there was usually low voltage in the RV septum, as was the case in this patient, although the area of low voltage was limited to the high RVOT, where there were matching pace maps for this particular VT. The VT was successfully ablated there (**Figure 28.3**).

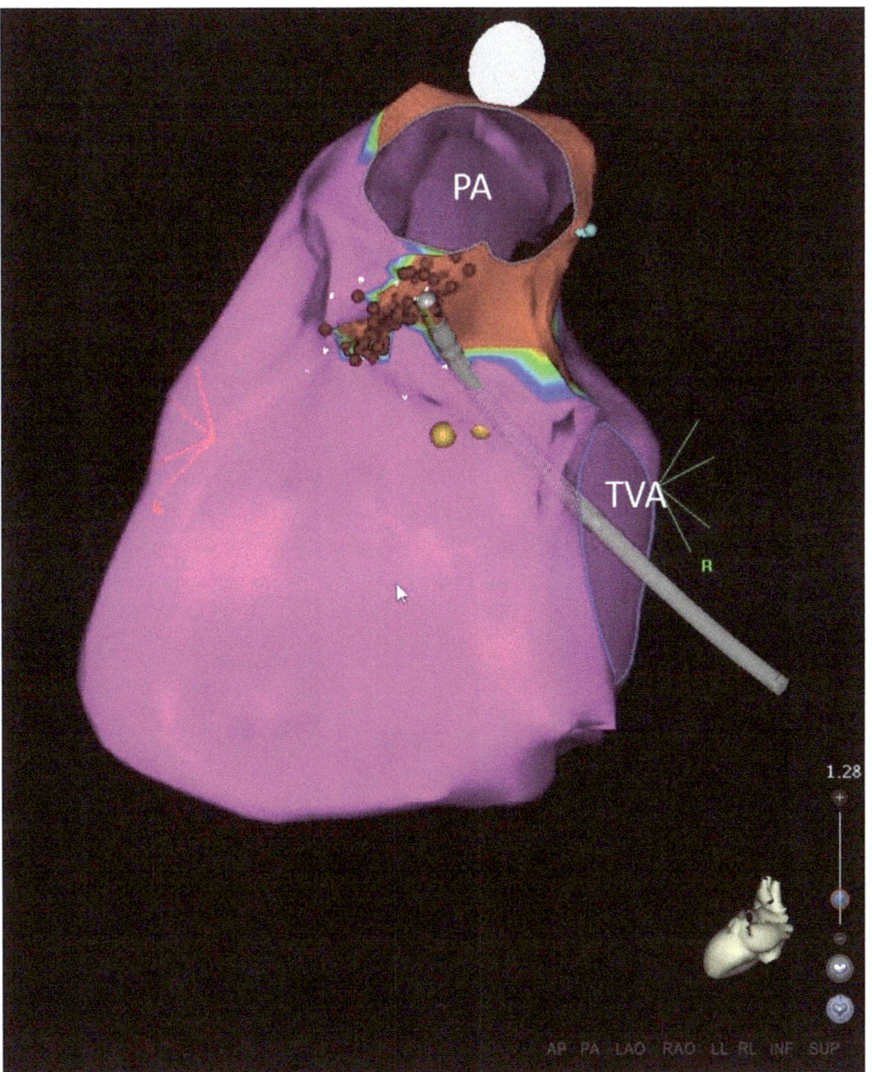

Figure 28.3 Electroanatomic bipolar voltage map of the septal RV. The catheter is in contact with a low-voltage area where the best pace map for this VT was located. Pace maps in the left ventricle did not show any matching pace maps. Pulmonary artery and tricuspid valve annulus are labeled.

REFERENCE

1. Yokokawa M, Good E, Crawford T, et al. Value of right ventricular mapping in patients with postinfarction ventricular tachycardia. *Heart Rhythm.* 2012;9:938–942.

CLINICAL HISTORY

A 53-year-old woman presented with frequent, symptomatic PVCs and a PVC burden of 26%. The patient had prior failed ablation procedures. She has a preserved left ventricular ejection fraction of 60%. She has a bicuspid aortic valve with mild aortic stenosis.

Question

Where does the PVC shown in **Figure 29.1** originate?

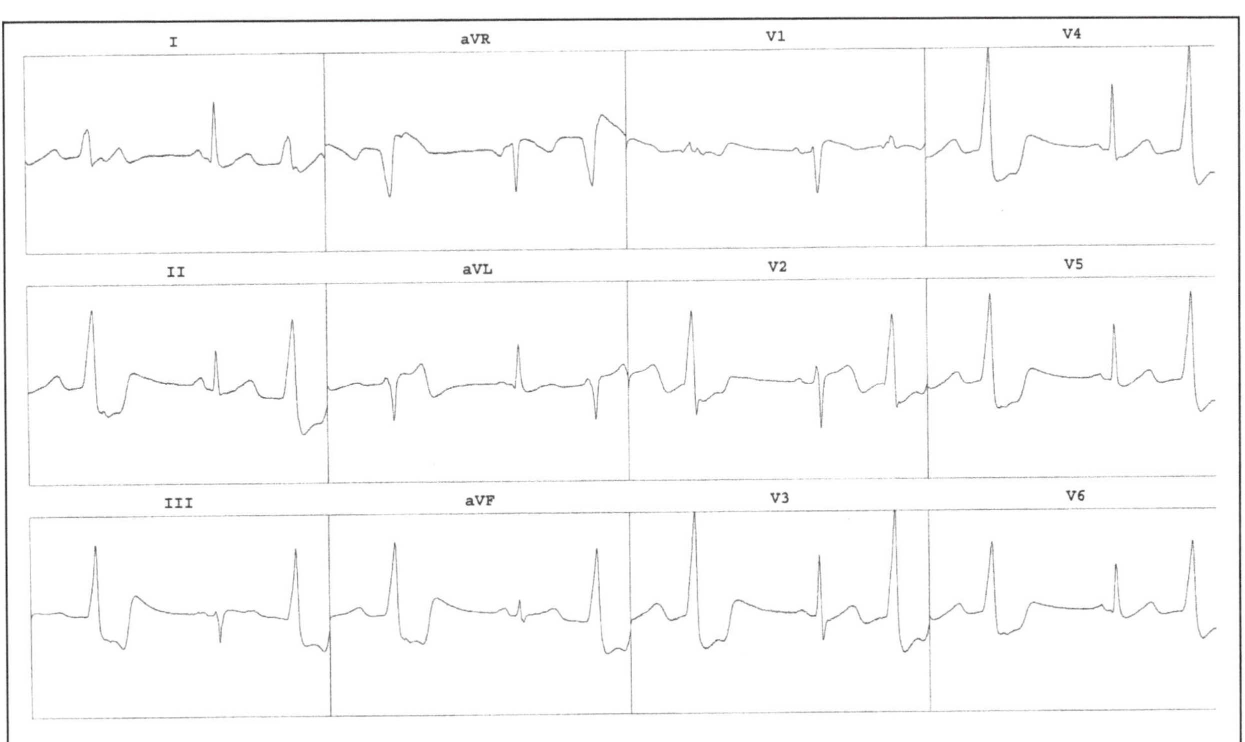

Figure 29.1   A 12-lead ECG with bigeminal PVC pattern.

Answer

The origin is from the commissure between the anterior and posterior leaflets of the aortic cusp in the setting of a bicuspid aortic valve. The patient had three prior procedures that failed to eliminate her arrhythmias. The ECG features suggestive of a cusp origin include early transition ($\leq V_3$), broad R wave (> 50% of QRS in V_1 or V_2), and R/S ratio > 30% in V_1 or V_2.[1] A QS or QR pattern in V_1 or V_2 would suggest an origin from the aortic commissure.[2,3] When looking at the described criterion of Q-wave amplitude aVL > aVR to distinguish supravalvular from infravalvular

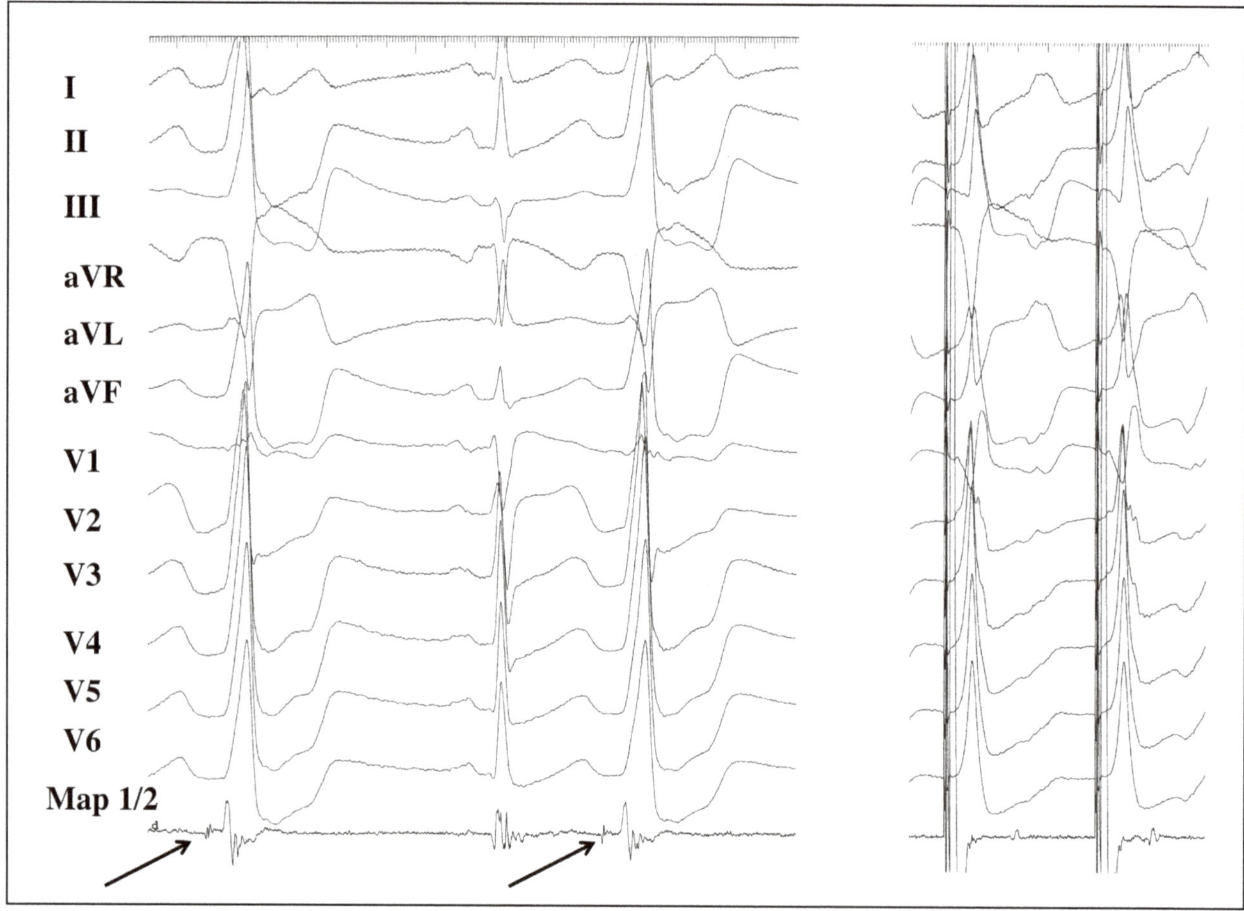

Figure 29.2   **Left panel:** Intracardiac tracings from the mapping catheter at the commissure between anterior and posterior cusps. An arrow indicates the earliest timing at the commissure. **Right panel:** Pace map at the site showing the prepotential in the left panel. There is no matching pace map.

arrhythmias, this would indicate a supravalvular origin.[4] Ablation was carried out in the commissure, but PVCs could not be eliminated permanently. The pace map from the earliest site where a prepotential was present (arrow in **Figure 29.2**) did not match with the spontaneous PVC, indicating a deeper intramural origin. Therefore, mapping was performed at the opposite RVOT that was about 5 mm from the commissure, and RF energy was delivered there (**Figure 29.3** and **Figure 29.4**). Although the pace map was very different, and the activation timing much later, ablation there eliminated the PVCs permanently.

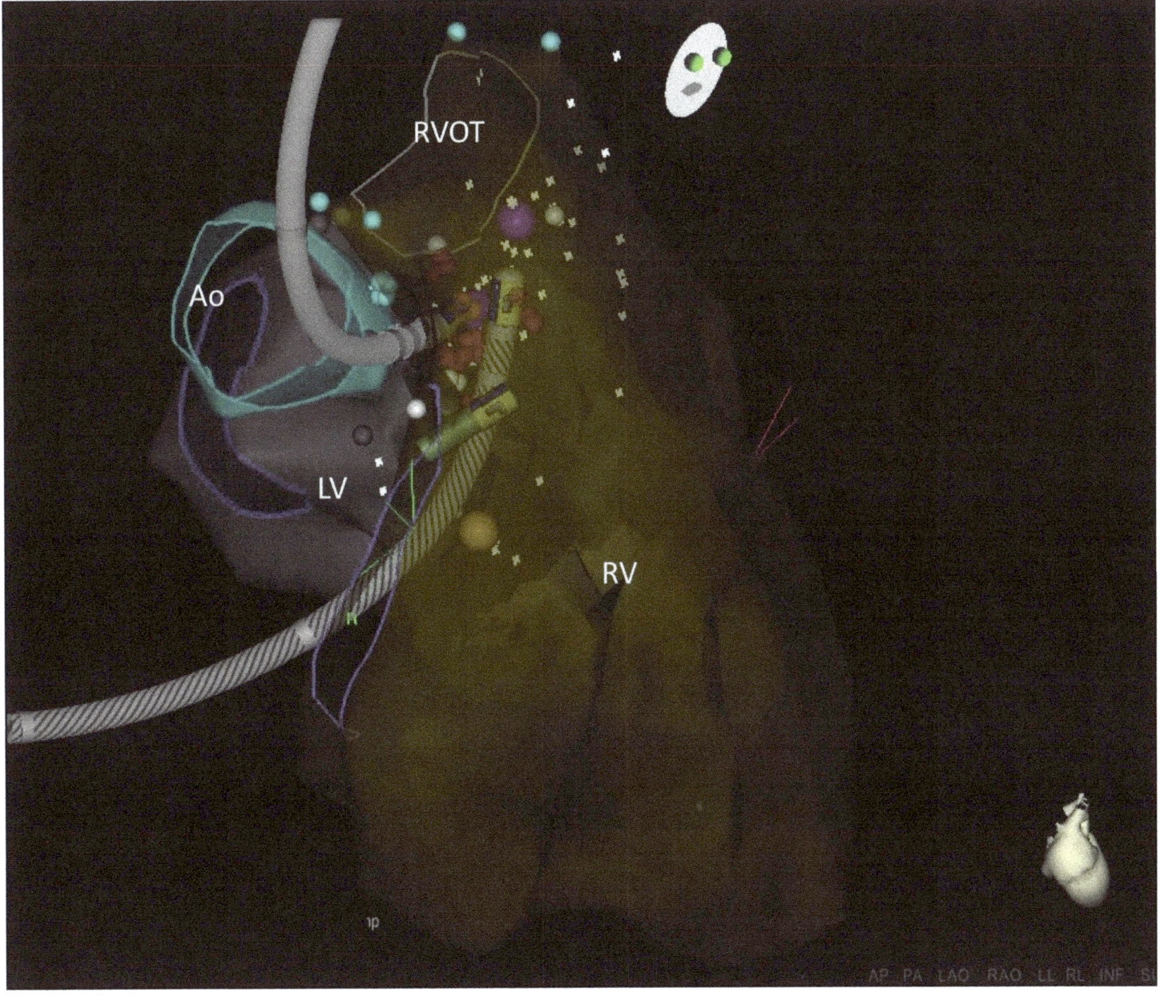

Figure 29.3 A 3D reconstruction of echocardiographic shells of the left ventricle (LV), the right ventricle (RV), and the aortic valve (Ao) with a catheter located in the aortic cusps, and the RVOT, where ablation was performed sequentially.

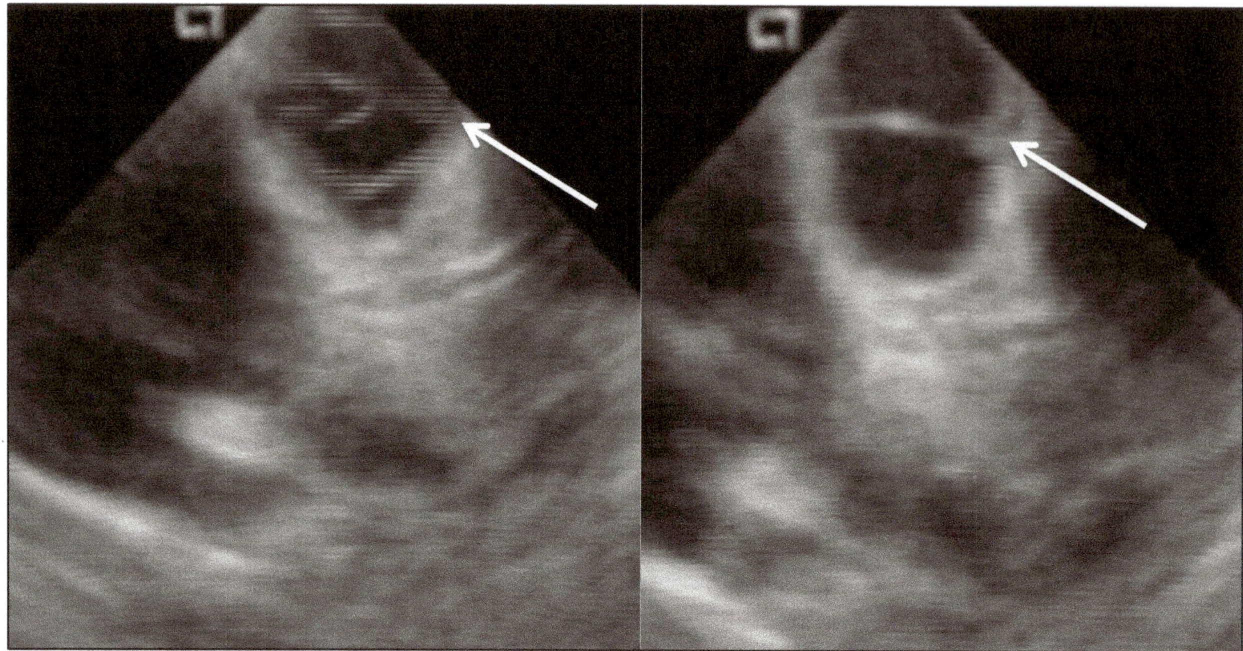

Figure 29.4 **Left panel:** Bicuspid aortic valve in open position. **Right panel:** Bicuspid aortic valve in closed position. **White arrows** indicate the site with early timing at the commissure separating anterior from posterior cusps.

REFERENCES

1. Ouyang F, Fotuhi P, Ho SY, et al. Repetitive monomorphic ventricular tachycardia originating from the aortic sinus cusp: Electrocardiographic characterization for guiding catheter ablation. *J Am Coll Cardiol.* 2002;39:500–508.
2. Bala R, Garcia FC, Hutchinson MD, et al. Electrocardiographic and electrophysiologic features of ventricular arrhythmias originating from the right/left coronary cusp commissure. *Heart Rhythm.* 2010;7:312–322.
3. Yamada T, Yoshida N, Murakami Y, et al. Electrocardiographic characteristics of ventricular arrhythmias originating from the junction of the left and right coronary sinuses of valsalva in the aorta: The activation pattern as a rationale for the electrocardiographic characteristics. *Heart Rhythm.* 2008;5:184–192.
4. Ouyang F, Mathew S, Wu S, et al. Ventricular arrhythmias arising from the left ventricular outflow tract below the aortic sinus cusps: Mapping and catheter ablation via transseptal approach and electrocardiographic characteristics. *Circ Arrhythm Electrophysiol.* 2014;7:445–455.

CLINICAL HISTORY

A 63-year-old man presented with frequent, asymptomatic PVCs. His ejection fraction was 35%. There was mid-wall delayed enhancement in his cardiac MRI. The patient had persistent atrial fibrillation with adequate rate control. He was referred for a PVC ablation procedure.

Question

Where does the PVC shown in **Figure 30.1** originate?

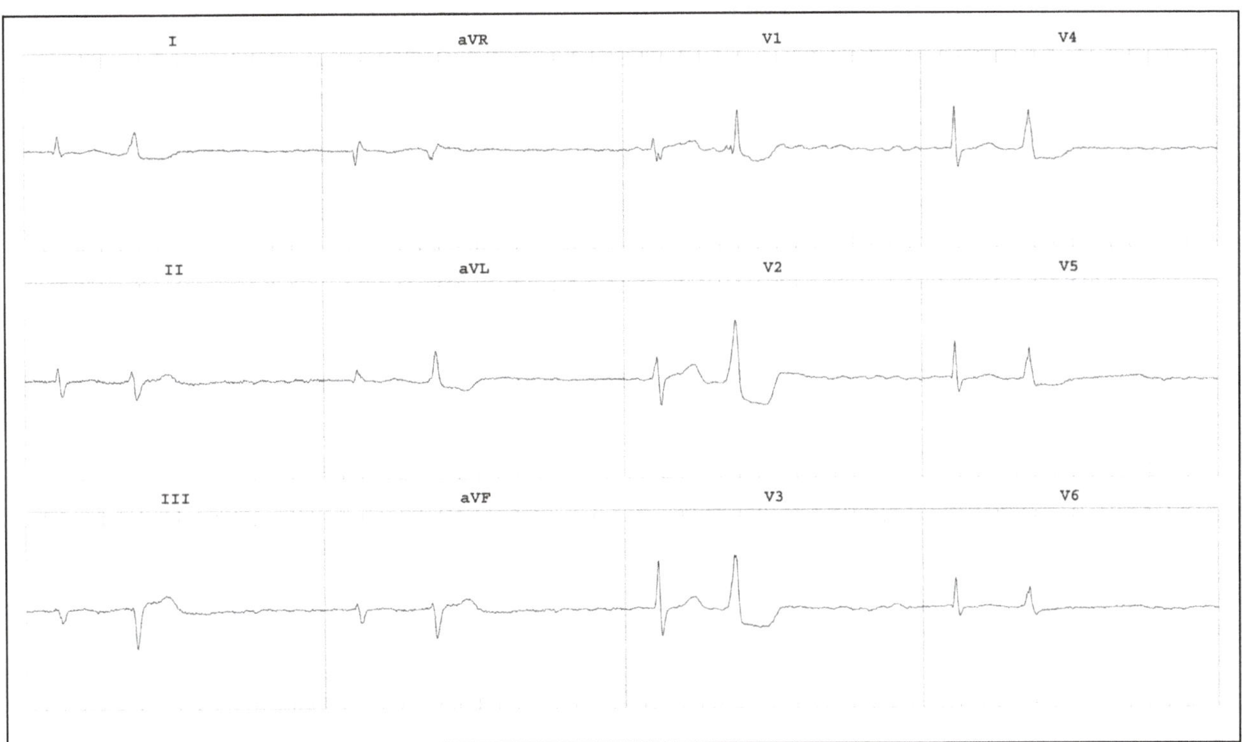

Figure 30.1   A 12-lead ECG with the patient's PVCs.

The origin is on the left inferior basal septum about 1 cm below the His bundle. There is positive concordance in the precordial leads indicating a basal origin. The axis is superior and indicates an inferior wall origin, combined with a relatively narrow QRS complex supporting a septal origin. The local activation time at the SOO was −45 ms with a matching pace map (**Figure 30.2**). The

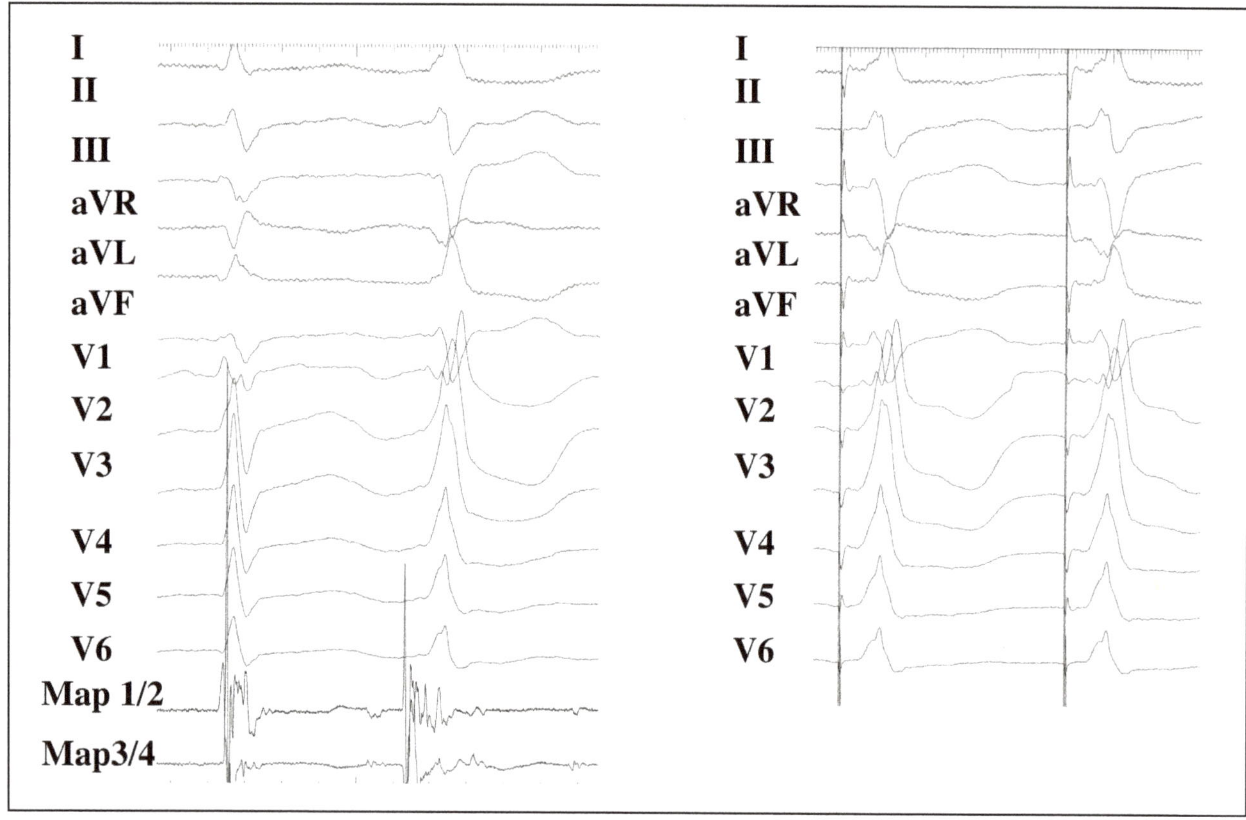

Figure 30.2   **Left panel:** Intracardiac tracings at the site of origin of the PVC. The presystolic activation time is −45 ms. **Right panel:** There is a matching pace map at this location.

SOO was at a safe distance to the His bundle, and ablation could be carried out without endangering AV nodal conduction (**Figure 30.3**). Of note, an inferior mitral annular origin does not always have positive concordance and therefore needs to be distinguished from papillary muscle origins where there is usually an R/S transition in leads V_3/V_4.

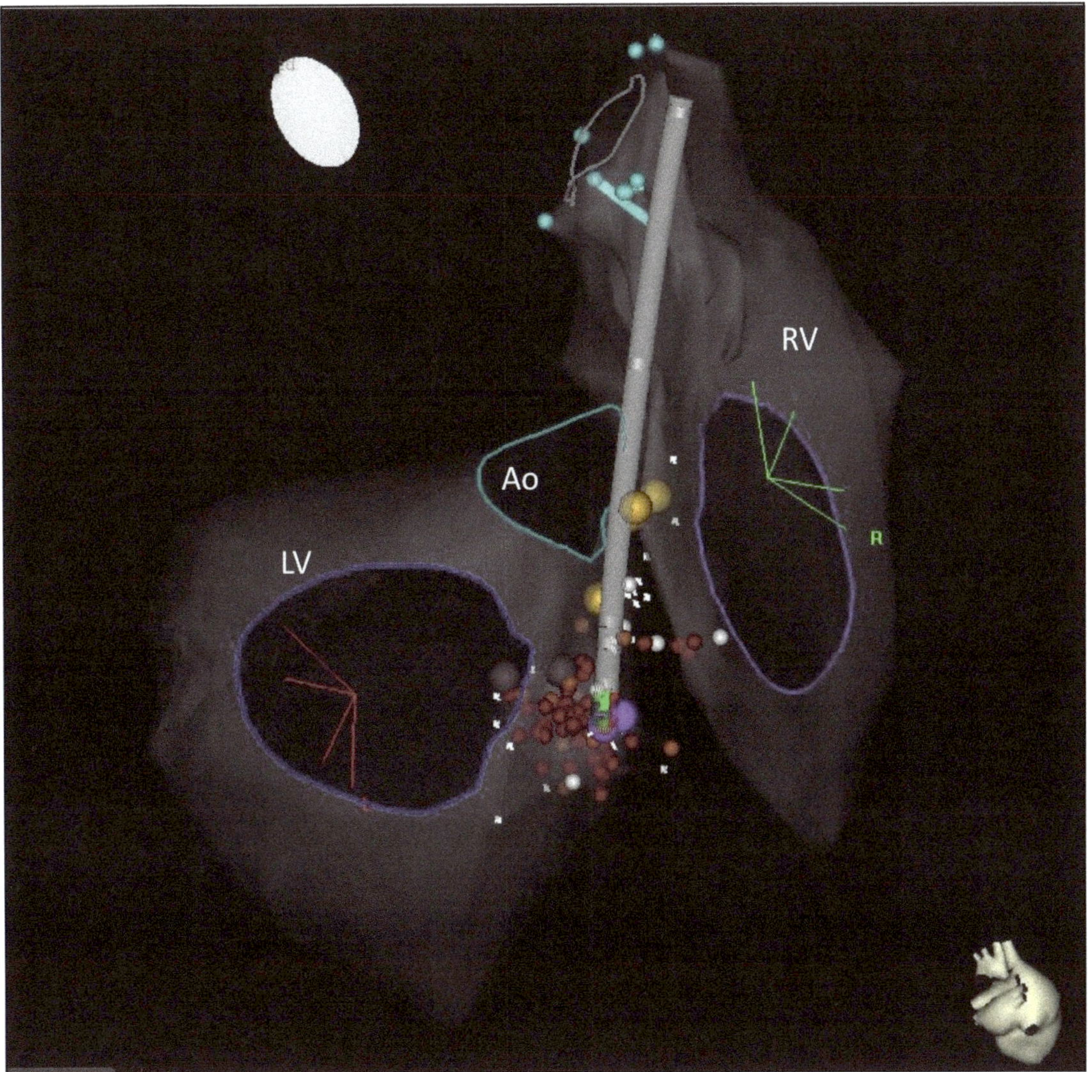

Figure 30.3 3D echocardiographic shells of the right and left ventricles (RV and LV) with the ablation catheter that is passed through the aortic valve (Ao) to the site of origin of the PVC, which is located about 1 cm inferior to the His bundle (**orange tag**).

Case 1: PVC originating from the anterior mitral valve annulus
Case 2: PVC originating from the posteroseptal tricuspid valve area
Case 3: PVC origin from the anterolateral papillary muscle
Case 4: VT originating from the anterior RVOT
Case 5: Bundle branch reentry VT
Case 6: VT originating from the anterior mitral valve annulus
Case 7: VT originating from the inferior tricuspid valve annulus
Case 8: VT originating from the anteroseptal RVOT
Case 9: PVC originating from the pulmonary artery
Case 10: VT originating from the posterior fascicle
Case 11: VT originating from scar involving the posterior fascicle
Case 12: VT originating from the epicardial inferior septum of the right ventricle
Case 13: PVC originating from the right bundle and the parahisian region
Case 14: PVC with intramural septal origin
Case 15: VT originating from the intramural scar
Case 16: PVC originating from the inferobasal epicardial right ventricle (crux of the heart)
Case 17: VT originating from the intramural septum
Case 18: VT originating from postinfarction scar
Case 19: PVC originating intrtamurally between RVOT and the R/L commissure of the aortic cusps
Case 20: PVC originating from an intramural scar
Case 21: PVC originating from the anterobasal left ventricular epicardium
Case 22: PVC originating from the commissure between right and left coronary cusp
Case 23: Couplets originating from the anteroapical left ventricle
Case 24: PVC originating from the slow pathway area
Case 25: PVC originating from an intramural focus
Case 26: VT originating from the septal aspect of the RVOT
Case 27: PVC originating from the LVOT
Case 28: VT originating from the interventricular septum
Case 29: PVC originating from the commissure betwenn anterior and posterior aortic cusp
Case 30: PVC originating from the LVOT below the His bundle

Printed in the USA
CPSIA information can be obtained
at www.ICGtesting.com
JSHW071917070224
56896JS00002B/3